PRACTICAL GUIDE TO HEALTH ASSESSMENT THROUGH THE LIFESPAN

This book features a new type of binding called otabind. When it is opened and the pages pressed down at the binding, the book will lie flat.

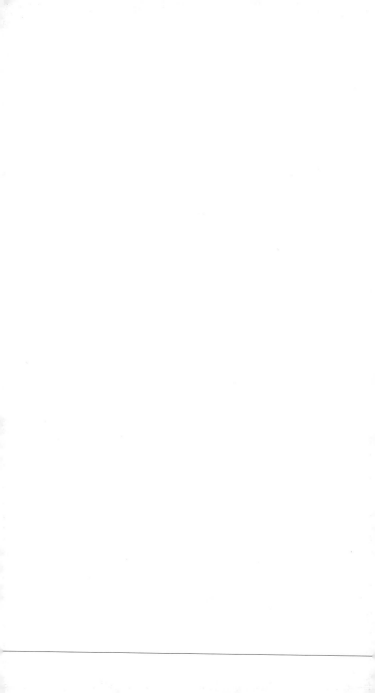

PRACTICAL GUIDE TO HEALTH ASSESSMENT THROUGH THE LIFESPAN

MILDRED O. HOGSTEL, Ph.D., R.N., C.
Abell-Hanger Professor of Gerontological Nursing
Harris College of Nursing
Texas Christian University
Fort Worth, Texas

RHONDA KEEN-PAYNE, Ph.D., R.N.
Associate Professor of Nursing
Harris College of Nursing
Texas Christian University
Fort Worth, Texas

With
Pediatric Adaptations by
LAURA YOUNG GIBSON, Ph.D., R.N., C.P.N.P.
Assistant Professor
School of Nursing
The University of Texas at Arlington
Arlington, Texas
and
Geriatric Adaptations by
MIRA KIRK NELSON, Ed.D., R.N., C.G.N.P.
Supervisor
Fort Worth City County Health Department
Fort Worth, Texas

F. A. DAVIS COMPANY ● Philadelphia

F. A. Davis Company
1915 Arch Street
Philadelphia, PA 19103

Printed in Canada

Last digit indicates print number: 10 9 8 7 6 5 4 3 2

nursing editor: Alan Sorkowitz
production editor: Gail Shapiro
cover design by: Steven R. Morrone

As new scientific information becomes available through basic and clinical research, recommended treatments and drug therapies undergo changes. The author(s) and publisher have done everything possible to make this book accurate, up to date, and in accord with accepted standards at the time of publication. The authors, editors, and publisher are not responsible for errors or omissions or for consequences from application of the book, and make no warranty, expressed or implied, in regard to the contents of the book. Any practice described in this book should be applied by the reader in accordance with professional standards of care used in regard to the unique circumstances that may apply in each situation. The reader is advised always to check product information (package inserts) for changes and new information regarding dose and contraindications before administering any drug. Caution is especially urged when using new or infrequently ordered drugs.

To
Our
Families
and
Students

Preface

Health assessment is an essential component of the nursing process and includes the health history, physical and mental status examinations, psychosocial history, and family and environmental assessment. The essential components of the assessment process may be completed in a few minutes in an emergency; at the other extreme, assessment may take place over several weeks in the client's home. The nurse has to use judgment in deciding which parts of the assessment are needed for a specific client in a certain setting.

The purpose of this book is to provide nursing students and practicing nurses in all settings with a practical and easy-to-use reference to the sequence and major components of health assessment. It is assumed that the user of this book will have completed courses in anatomy and physiology and completed or currently be enrolled in a complete course in health assessment.

This book can easily be kept in a pocket until needed. When the nurse is ready to perform any part of the assessment, the book may be placed on a table near the client's bed or chair. The book has been designed for rapid reference. When the book is opened and the pages pressed down at the binding, they will lie flat, and they can easily be read at a distance, thus freeing the nurse's hands for the assessment. Because the book is meant to be practical and useful, only essential information has been included. The equipment needed, sequence, and techniques for each system are presented as succinctly as possible, often accompanied by relevant diagrams or illustrations. The steps of what to assess in carrying out a physical examination of each body system are listed. It should be noted that some of the assessment techniques, for example, an internal gynecological examination and a prostate examination, are included as essential components of a total assessment but they will not be performed by the novice practitioner.

Normal and/or *common* findings and *significant deviations* from normal are included for each system. *Common* findings are those that are not considered *normal* because they do not occur in everyone but that rarely need referral (for example, lentigo senilis in older adults or cradle cap in infants). *Common* and *significant* findings that should be referred for follow-up are shown in red. A special section, clinical alert, is also in red. This section notes special instructions the nurse needs to be aware of during the assessment and/or concerns related to the findings.

A few sample diagnostic tests are listed for each system. The nurse will refer the client to a physician, nurse practitioner (where appropriate), or other health care provider who may order and evaluate the diagnostic tests. Sample North American Nursing Diagnosis Association (NANDA) nursing diagnoses are also included for each system. These are not meant to be inclusive because nursing diagnoses are very individualized. However, the samples should guide the reader toward other possible diagnoses. These diagnoses should be helpful in preparing individual care plans after the assessment phase. Essential patient/family education and home health notes for each system also are included.

Pediatric and geriatric adaptations have been added for each section of the health history, physical examination, and patient/family education. For each body system a brief sample of how to document the physical findings is presented. Samples of primarily *normal* and some *common abnormal* findings are documented. *Significant deviations* from normal will need more detailed documentation. These samples are only a general guide, because methods of documentation vary with the format, setting, and the client's needs or status.

A glossary of the most commonly used abbreviations and terms in health assessment appears at the back of the book so that other references will not be needed for this information. The Appendices contain selected sample history and physical assessment forms. Following them is a list of health assessment texts that may be consulted for further reading, if necessary.

The authors believe that nurses will find this assessment book a helpful, time-saving clinical guide while learning or becoming more skilled in health assessment techniques in the classroom or any clinical setting in which they assess patients.

Mildred O. Hogstel
Rhonda Keen-Payne

Acknowledgments

The authors express their appreciation to Sam Sanders, former Coordinator of the Learning Resource Center, Harris College of Nursing, Texas Christian University, Fort Worth, Texas, for drawing some of the illustrations for this publication; to Esther Ochoa, Secretary, to Susan Moore, Administrative Assistant, for typing the manuscript, and to Terry Sheridan, Secretary, for the many small ways she has assisted in preparation of the manuscript.

Consultants

Esther Acree, RN, MSN, FNP
Assistant Professor
Indiana State University
School of Nursing
Terre Haute, Indiana

Marian A. Conway, RN, C, MSN
Assistant Professor
Armstrong State College
Department of Baccalaureate Nursing
Savannah, Georgia

Donna M. Fair, RN, MSN
Assistant Professor of Adult Nursing
Medical College of Georgia
Augusta, Georgia

Marilyn Rhoads, RN, MSN
Assistant Professor
School of Nursing
Austin Peay State University
Clarksville, Tennessee

Colleen Smitherman, PhD, RN
Associate Professor
Kirkhof School of Nursing
Grand Valley State University
Allendale, Michigan

Nancy Burk Williamson, PhD, RN
Medical College of Georgia
School of Nursing
Augusta, Georgia

Contents

List of Figures

List of Tables

PART 1

The Client Interview and Health History

Review of Nursing Process

This book will focus on the assessment phase of the nursing process. Specific nursing diagnoses can be determined only after a thorough assessment of an individual patient or client. Refer to Appendix A for a list of the most current approved NANDA nursing diagnoses.

FIVE MAJOR COMPONENTS

1. Assessment
   a. Subjective data
      (1) Nursing history (patient and family)
   b. Objective data
      (1) Physical findings
      (2) Laboratory and diagnostic test results
2. Nursing Diagnosis
   a. Problems identified and solvable by the nurse
3. Planning
   a. Patient goals
   b. Expected outcomes (short-term goals)
   c. Long-term goals
   d. Nursing orders
4. Intervention
   a. Implementation of the plan
   b. Nursing action
   c. Discharge planning/teaching

5. Evaluation
   a. Evaluation of the patient goals and expected outcomes
   b. Additional assessment
   c. Addition or revision of nursing diagnoses
   d. Revision of goals, expected outcomes, and nursing orders

Health History Guidelines

(See Appendix B for a sample health history form.)

TIPS FOR INTERVIEWING

- Sit if possible (relaxes the client) so that the client can see your lips.
- Attend to client comfort first.
- Establish eye contact (shows genuine concern) unless inappropriate because of ethnic background of client.
- Listen attentively (clarify when needed).
- Avoid unnecessary medical jargon.
- Look and listen for cues (e.g., changes in facial expression or posture) for follow-up questions.
- Ask nonleading open-ended questions.
- Use an amplifying device (stethoscope or other assistive device) for persons with decreased hearing function.
- Complete in less than 20 minutes if in an acute care setting.

INFORMATION NEEDED FOR A COMPLETE HEALTH HISTORY*

Date of History

Personal Data

- Name
- Sex

---

*Adapted from Nelson, M. and Mayfield, P.: Health assessment. In Hogstel, M. (ed.): *Nursing Care of the Older Adult,* 2nd ed. John Wiley & Sons, New York, 1988, pp. 119–128.

- DOB
- Place of birth
- Age
- Ethnic background
- Marital status
- Address
- Phone number
- Name of physician
- Social Security number
- Medicare number/Medicaid number
- Other insurance name and number
- Religious preference, including church or synagogue membership
- Person to be contacted in an emergency (name, address, phone number)
- Education
- Occupation

Reason for Seeking Health Care (Chief Complaint [CC])

History of Present Illness (PI)

- Onset
- What evokes?
- What relieves?
- Manifestations
- Treatment
- Complications

Past Health History

- Client's perception of level of health in general
- Childhood illnesses
- Genogram (family history of diseases)
- Immunizations
- Allergies
- Serious accidents/injuries
- Major adult illnesses
- Behavioral problems
- Surgical procedures

- Other hospitalizations
- Obstetric history
- Environmental hazards
  ◦ Home
  ◦ Work
  ◦ Community
- Blood transfusions

Current Medications

- Prescription medications
- Client's understanding of reasons medications were prescribed
- OTC preparations
- Home remedies
- Borrowed medications

Personal Habits and Patterns of Living

- Work. Type, length of time employed, stresses
- Rest/sleep. How much, when, aids
- Exercise/ambulation. How much, when, aids
- Recreation/leisure/hobbies. Type, amount
- Nutrition. Time, foods, fluids, and amounts for all meals (24-hour recall) and snacks; recent changes in appetite; special diet
- Caffeine. Source, amount
- Alcohol/other drugs. Type, number of years used, amount, perceived problems with level of use
- Tobacco. Type, number of years used, amount per day
- Urinary/bowel activity. Frequency, amount, problems
- Sexual activity. Level of activity, use of contraceptives, problems, sexual preference, sexual orientation

Activities of Daily Living. Note the client's ability to perform (alone or with help) the following activities:
- Ambulating
- Dressing

- Grooming
- Bathing
- Toileting
- Eating
- Using the telephone
- Doing laundry
- Housekeeping
- Obtaining access to the community
- Driving
- Food purchasing
- Food preparation

Psychosocial History

Inquire about and document the following:
- Significant others, relationship, proximity
- Support system
- Typical 24-hour weekday and weekend day
- Living arrangements
  ○ Number of rooms
  ○ Number and ages of other individuals in home
- Significant stressors
- Coping ability
- Feelings about self (self-concept, functional status, adaptations, independence, body image, sexuality, sexual orientation)
- History of interpersonal trauma (rape, incest, abuse as child or spouse). Note ability to discuss, stage in resolution (denial, fear, anger, grief, adaptation), resources
- Understanding of and feelings about current illness
- Psychological problems

Mental Status Assessment

- Appearance (dress, hygiene, mannerisms, gestures)
- Eye contact

- Position, posture, gait
- Orientation
  - Person (first and last name)
  - Place (name of facility or home address)
  - Time (year, month, date of month, day of week, season, A.M. or P.M.)
- Speech (volume, clarity, speed, quantity, tone, accent)
- Affect (alert, calm, responsive)
- Mood (sad, depressed, joyful)
- Memory (immediate, recent, remote)
- Intelligence (vocabulary, calculations)
- Abstract thinking (judgment, proverbs, analogies)
- Attention span (limited)
- Thought content (depression, paranoid beliefs, obsessions, hallucinations, phobias, delusions, illusions)
- Thought process (logical, spontaneous, flight of ideas, bizarre, tangential)
- Insight (awareness and meaning of illness)
- Attitude (cooperative, evasive, passive, hostile)
- Activity level (appropriate, restless, lethargic)

NOTE

1. See Sample Mental Status Assessment Flow Sheet (Hogstel, 1991) in Appendix D.
2. See Short Portable Mental Status Questionnaire (SPMSQ) (Pfiffer, 1975) in Appendix E.

Review of Systems

See Part 3, ''Body Organ and System Assessment,'' for specific questions to ask about each system.

- General
- Integument (skin, hair, nails)
- Head
- Eyes
- Ears
- Nose and sinuses

- Mouth and throat
- Neck
- Lungs and thorax
- Breasts and axillae
- Cardiovascular
- Abdomen
- Musculoskeletal
- Male genitalia and rectum
- Female genitalia and rectum
- Neurologic
- Adaptations in pregnancy

Pediatric Additions to the Health History

PERSONAL DATA

- Child's nickname
- Parents' telephone numbers (home and work)

REASON FOR SEEKING HEALTH CARE (CC)

- Person who wanted the child to see a health care provider (child, parent, teacher)

HISTORY OF PI

- Parents' reaction to child's illness
- What the child gains and loses from seeking health care

PAST HEALTH HISTORY

Mother's Health During Pregnancy

- Age
- Any drugs taken (prescription, nonprescription, alcohol, illegal drugs)
- Planned pregnancy?
- Complications

- Illnesses
- Concerns
- Exposure to toxins or other hazards (radon, chemicals)

Natal History

- Length of gestation
- Location of birth
- Type of labor (induced, spontaneous; < 12 hours, > 24 hours) and delivery (spontaneous, forceps, cesarean; anesthesia)
- Apgar scores (see Appendix F)
- Birth weight
- Complications

Neonatal History

- Congenital anomalies
- Condition of infant
- Oxygen use
- Estimation of gestational age
- Problems (feeding, jaundice, respiratory distress)
- Age at discharge from hospital
- Weight at discharge from hospital
- First month of life (family adaptations, responses to baby, perceived ability of family to care for baby)

Infant and Childhood History

- Illnesses. Note exposure, specific disorders, residual effects.
- Allergies (eczema, allergic rhinitis, hives, vomiting after introduction of new foods, diarrhea)
- Immunizations. Note each vaccine, age when received, reactions.
- Screening tests. Note types and the child's age when each test was performed (vision, hearing, scoliosis, sickle cell anemia).

- Operations/hospitalizations. Note the child's and parents' reactions to the events.
- Accident/trauma history. Note consistency of explanations and emotional response to questioning if abuse is suspected.

Feeding History

- Feedings/supplements (type, amount)
- Weight gain
- Age at which solid foods started
- Type of solid foods fed
- Infant's responses to foods
- Parents' responses to feeding their infant
- Weaning
- Food preferences
- Current feeding (type, schedules)
- Ability to feed self

Developmental History

Note the child's height and weight at different ages, as well as the age when the child was able to:

- Hold head up
- Roll over
- Reach for toys
- Sit alone
- Crawl
- Stand alone
- Walk
- Say first word
- Talk in two-word sentences
- Dress self
- Use the toilet (urination, bowel movement)

SEXUAL DEVELOPMENT, EDUCATION, AND ACTIVITY

- Present status of sexual development
- Age of voice changes and pubic hair growth (males)

- Age of breast development and menarche (females)
- Social relations with same and opposite sex
- Curiosity about sexuality
- Masturbation
- Contraception
- Parental responses and instructions to the child about sexuality and dating
- Child's use of language to discuss sexuality. Note age appropriateness and indicators of precocity. Note behaviors suggestive of sexual abuse.

SOCIAL HISTORY

- Sleep. Patterns, problems, terrors
- Speech (stuttering, delays)
- Habits (rocking, nail biting)
- Discipline used. Type, frequency, effectiveness, attitudes, response of parents to temper tantrums
- School. Current grade, any preschool attendance, adjustments, failures, favorite subjects, performance, problems
- Social behavior. Relationships with peers, parents, authority figures; type of peer group, level of independence; interests/hobbies; self-image. If infant, toddler, or preschooler, note child-parent interactions, demonstration of affection, willingness of child to separate from parent (least likely age 8–20 months), evidence of increasing independence and competence.

FAMILY HISTORY

- Maternal gestational history
- Any consanguinity in family
- Employment history
- Child care arrangements
- Adequacy of clothing, food, transportation, sleep arrangements
- Parents' relationship to each other

- Parents' illnesses
- Siblings' relationship to each other
- Siblings' illnesses

Geriatric Additions to the Health History

IMMUNIZATIONS

- Pneumonia vaccine (dates)
- Influenza vaccine (date of last immunization)
- Tetanus (date of last administration)

CURRENT PRESCRIPTION MEDICATIONS

- Names of the medications
- Prescribing health care professional(s)
- Prescribed dosages and whether the client is overdosing or underdosing
- Side effects
- Adherence problems
- Visual difficulties related to medications
- Ability to afford the medications
- Ability to get to the pharmacy
- Difficulty swallowing or administering drugs
- Client's opinion of drug efficacy
- Borrowed medications, if any
- Understanding of total medication regimen (purpose, method, time, action, dose, side effects, interactions)

CURRENT OTC MEDICATIONS

- Names of the medications
- Dosages (amount, frequency)
- Reasons for taking
- Side effects
- Home remedies, folk medicine

NUTRITION

- Salt and sugar intake. Note whether the client adds salt or sugar to food at the table or in cooking; the amount of sugar used on cereal and in coffee/tea; other food items with high salt or sugar content.
- Weight. Note any weight changes (up or down) in the client over the past month, 1 year, or 5 years. Client's perception of weight.
- Special diet. If the client follows a special diet, note the type and any difficulty adhering to the diet. Assess knowledge of diet.
- Food preferences. Note client's current food likes/dislikes, amounts of food consumed at one time, frequency of meals, typical meals.
- Appetite. Note whether the client's hunger is more pronounced at certain times of the day or night; any loss of or increase in appetite recently or over the past year.
- Food purchase and preparation. Note who buys and prepares the food, and whether the client likes it; if client prepares own food, note whether preparation is a problem. If so, is problem due to fatigue, eating alone, decreased vision, difficulty using the refrigerator or stove?
- Ingestion. Note any difficulty the client has in feeding self, chewing, or swallowing.
- Affordability. Note whether the client is able to afford the food needed and desired.

ACTIVITIES OF DAILY LIVING

Note whether the client requires any assistance in:
- Dressing (fastening buttons, zippers; tying shoes)
- Trimming fingernails or toenails, shaving, brushing teeth, brushing hair
- Bathing in the tub or shower (preparing bath water, getting into/out of the tub or shower, washing all body parts)
- Using the toilet

- Ambulating in the home (getting into/out of bed, lowering into/getting up from chairs, walking, climbing stairs, reaching for items in cupboards, opening doors)
- Eating (handling utensils, cutting food, putting food into mouth)
- Doing laundry, either by hand or with a washing machine
- Planning, preparing, and serving adequate meals independently
- Housekeeping (making the bed, cleaning the house, washing dishes, taking out the garbage)

Note whether the client has access to transportation (bus, car) for shopping, going to the doctor.

If the client needs assistance with any activities, explore further the extent of help required. Is help available?

Family Assessment

Inquire about and document the following:

- Spouse (age, health status, length of marriage, cause of death if deceased)
- Children/grandchildren/great-grandchildren (number, ages, health status, cause of deaths if deceased)
- Siblings/parents/grandparents/great grandparents (ages, health status, cause of deaths if deceased)
- Family illnesses (past and present)
- Recent changes in family structure (divorce, adoption, remarriage, death)
- Members of current household (related and not related)
- Family members who make major decisions about the family
- Family relationships (roles, conflicts)
- Ethnic/cultural background and traditions related to health
- Family activities (social, religious, vacations, recreation)
- Economic resources and concerns
- Usual health providers (MD, DO, NP)
- Pets (type, number, meaning to the family)

Environmental Assessment

HOSPITAL OR NURSING HOME

- Observe the client's facial expression and posture in bed.
- Note the placement and position of the bed.
- Check the bed and bed rails for proper functioning and position.
- Assess any equipment attached to the client and/or bed (NG tubing, urinary catheter, IV, monitor) for proper functioning.
- Make sure that the call cord, the telephone, paper wipes, and water (if allowed) are within easy reach of the client.
- Note whether privacy and space for the client's personal possessions are adequate.
- Note any unusual odors emanating from the client or in the room.
- Note whether the floor is free from litter and moisture.
- Make sure no unnecessary equipment and/or supplies are in the room.

HOME*

- Neighborhood location (urban, suburban, rural)
- Sidewalks, paved streets, presence of churches, schools, playgrounds, industries/businesses
- Traffic patterns in neighborhood
- Size and type of home (apartment, house, trailer)
- Description of the home
- Whether client owns or rents the home
- Length of time in current home
- Distance to shopping
- Type of water supply
- Type of sewage disposal
- Type and efficiency of heating and cooling systems

---

*Adapted with permission from Browning, M.: Guide for assessment of home environment. In Hogstel, M. (ed.): *Nursing Care of the Older Adult,* 2nd ed. John Wiley & Sons, New York, 1988, pp. 533–537.

- Type of transportation (car, bus, walking)
- Presence of a telephone or emergency signaling system
- Neighbors (proximity; whether client perceives as supportive or threatening)
- Adequacy of lighting outside and inside, including night lights
- Distance to streetlights, fire hydrant, fire station
- Visibility of path from car to house by neighbors
- Safety of the inside and outside stairs, number of steps
- Security of the outside doors
- Activities of neighborhood residents: Note children at play outdoors, transient persons, older residents' visibility, activity after dark.
- Client's perception of safety for self in environment. Note client's awareness of crimes in area, perception of own vulnerability; degree to which precautions/fear affects daily activities.
- Presence, placement, and functioning of smoke alarms
- Presence and placement of fire extinguishers
- Safety of the bathroom floor, tub, commode; functioning of the fixtures
- Temperature of the hot water $\leq 120°F$
- Condition of the floors and stairs (cleanliness, evenness, freedom from clutter, presence of throw rugs)
- Safety and state of repair of the furniture
- Safe use of appliances and electrical cords
- Functioning refrigerator, stove
- Presence of books, radio, television, newspaper, magazines
- Proper storage of household cleaners
- Proper storage of food and medicines
- Availability of laundry facilities
- Availability and functioning of lawn equipment
  Summary at end of total health history
  Ask whether there is anything else that the client would like
to tell or ask you.

PART 2

The Physical Examination

Physical Examination Guidelines

(See Appendix C for a sample physical assessment form.)

PREPARATION GUIDELINES

- Provide a warm, comfortable, private environment with natural lighting, if possible.
- Eliminate distractions and disruptions.
- Check all needed equipment for proper functioning and place it within easy reach.
- Introduce yourself to the client by name and title.
- Have the client void before the examination; collect clean specimen if needed.
- Explain what you are going to do and why.
- Warm your hands and instruments before touching the client's skin.

Physical Examination Guidelines

- If right-handed, stand on the client's right side. Move to the client's back (for posterior thorax) and to the client's left side (for left eye), as needed. You should be able to circle the bed or table.
- Drape the client well, exposing only those areas that are being examined.

- Be aware of your nonverbal communication during the examination; avoid frightening, intimidating, or embarrassing the client.
- Warn the client when any part of the examination may be uncomfortable.
- Be as gentle as possible.
- Be especially careful when examining sensitive areas (eyes, breasts, genitals).
- Always wear gloves when you may come in contact with *any* body fluids or open lesion.
- Carefully assess those areas where potential problems or concerns were discovered in the history and review of systems.

TECHNIQUES IN PHYSICAL ASSESSMENT

Inspection

- Requires good lighting (preferably daylight rather than artificial light) and full exposure of area
- Systematically observe color, size, shape, symmetry, position. Note any impairment of function.

Auscultation

- Use stethoscope diaphragm for bowel, breath, and cardiac sounds. Use bell for vascular and cardiac sounds.
- Assess for loudness, pitch, quality or nature, frequency, and duration.

Percussion (see Fig. 1)

- Requires knowledge of anatomic location of internal organs and their approximate size
- Indirect method:
  Place middle finger only of nondominant hand on area to be percussed. Using the tip of the middle finger of dominant hand, strike the nondominant resting finger with a quick bouncing blow. Compare the sounds on the right and left

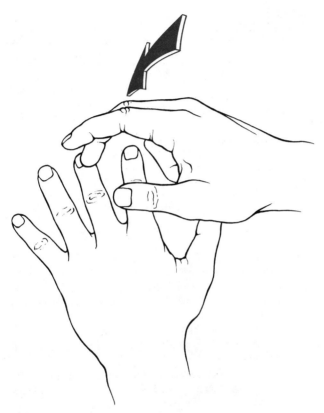

FIGURE 1.
Percussion technique.

sides of the body with each other and with Percussion Sounds Chart (see Table 1).

Palpation

- Requires touching with different parts of hand and with varying pressures to determine characteristics of pain, temperature, size, shape, moisture and/or texture.

TABLE 1
PERCUSSION SOUNDS

Tone	Characteristics	Possible Source
Tympanic	Loud, clear, drumlike	Low density, such as abdominal distention with gas
Resonant	Hollow, loud	Mixed density, such as healthy lung
Hyperresonant	Echoing, hollow	Mixed density, such as emphysematous lung
Dull	Quiet, thudding	High density, such as liver
Flat	Quiet, short, flat	High density, such as bone, thick muscle

- Explain touch to patient. Warm hands.
- Use light palpation before deep palpation.
- Use pads of fingers to identify texture, size, shape, movement (e.g., pulse).
- Use dorsum of fingers for temperature assessment.
- Gently pinch skin to assess turgor on forehead or upper third of sternum.
- Use palms or ulnar side of hand to assess vibrations.
- Use deep palpation gently and briefly to assess areas such as pelvis and abdomen for body organs and masses.
- Palpate areas of pain last.

Pediatric Adaptations

GENERAL GUIDELINES

- If the child does not know you, it is best if there is someone else in the room whom the child trusts, preferably a parent or other family member.
- Parents can assist by telling you how they cope with the child.

SUGGESTIONS FOR SPECIFIC AGE GROUPS

Younger Infants

- Let the parent assist by holding the child on his or her lap.

Older Infants

- Parents should be within the child's view.
- Move slowly and approach the child slowly.
- Restrain the child adequately and gently with parents' assistance.

Toddlers and Preschoolers

- Keep the parents in the room, ask them to assist when appropriate.
- Tell the child it is all right to cry or yell.
- Allow the child to play with the equipment if desired (during the history taking).
- Use distraction.
- Perform the nonthreatening parts of the examination first.
- Use a doll to demonstrate certain parts of the examination.
- Restrain the child adequately.
- Use the parents to assist (e.g., holding stethoscope on the child's chest).
- Give the child simple choices when possible.

Preschoolers

- Explain briefly what the child will experience.
- Demonstrate the equipment, allow the child to play with it, or use it on a doll.
- Let the child know that the examination is not punishment.
- Involve the child by allowing him or her to hold the chart or stethoscope for you.
- Praise the child for helping and cooperating.

School-aged Children

- Explain the examination and allow time for questions.
- Explain what you are doing.
- Allow the child to assist by handing equipment to you.
- Allow the child to listen, feel, or see what you find.
- Protect the child's privacy.

Adolescents

- Explain the examination and encourage questions.
- Examine the child apart from parents and ask if there are any questions.
- Tell the child the findings and the norms (e.g., ''Your breasts are beginning to develop; that is normal for a 12-year-old'').
- Protect the child's privacy.

Geriatric Adaptations

GENERAL GUIDELINES

- Allow ample time for examining the client because older people move more slowly and take longer to react and respond to questions.
- To avoid chilling, keep the client warmly covered, exposing each body part only briefly.
- To conserve the client's energy, organize the examination to minimize position changes.
- Assist the client on and off the examining table and with position changes. (Older people are at greater risk of falling than younger ones.)

POSSIBLE MODIFICATIONS

- If the client has breathing problems or a curvature of the spine, it may be necessary to elevate the examining table and/or use pillows.
- If the client has a musculoskeletal disorder and/or feels dizzy, some neurologic tests may need to be omitted.

Suggested Sequence of the Health Examination

NOTE: The following sequence illustrates *one* method to integrate all systems for a complete examination at one time. This method focuses on efficiency of time and helps to protect and preserve the patient's energy.

HISTORY

OVERVIEW

- Vital signs (radial pulses), BP
- Height, weight
- Speech, cognition, mental status, interaction
- Gait, Romberg, coordination, balance

INTEGUMENT

(Client sitting)
- Inspect and palpate all visible skin surfaces.
- Evaluate lesions (draw if helpful).
- Inspect hair and nails.

HEAD

- Cranium
- Eyes, cranial nerves (CN) II, III, IV, V, VI
- Ears, CN VIII
- Nose, CN I
- Sinuses
- Mouth, CN XII
- Throat, CN IX
- Preauricular and postauricular and occipital nodes

NECK

- Carotid pulses
- Thyroid gland

- Lymph nodes
- Range of motion (ROM), CN XI
- Jugular veins

BACK

- Inspect, percuss, palpate, auscultate
- Fremitus, respiratory excursion
- Symmetry, spinal alignment
- Costovertebral angle tenderness
- Mobility

ANTERIOR TRUNK

(Client seated and/or lying)
- Inspect the breasts.
- Auscultate breath sounds, heart sounds, carotid pulses, apical impulse (compare rate of apical impulse with radial pulse).
- Assess ROM of upper extremities.
- Palpate brachial pulses.
- Palpate the breasts, axillary, and epitrochlear lymph nodes.
- Palpate thrills, PMI.
- With client on left side or leaning forward, auscultate apex for murmurs.

ABDOMEN

- Inspect movement, color, contour.
- Auscultate the four quadrants.
- Auscultate for bruits over abdominal aorta, renal artery, iliac artery, and femoral artery.
- Percuss the abdomen.
- Palpate the abdomen.
- Palpate/percuss for bladder distention.
- Measure the size of the liver.
- Palpate the inguinal nodes, femoral pulses.
- Assess ROM of remaining joints if the client is unable to stand.
- Palpate popliteal, dorsalis pedis, and posterior tibial pulses.

MUSCULOSKELETAL SYSTEM

- Extremities (check for edema).
- Inspect and palpate joints for tenderness, heat, crepitus.

NEUROLOGIC SYSTEM

- Assess color, warmth, strength, ROM, gait, gross motor movement.
- Test the reflexes: biceps, triceps, brachioradialis, patellar, achilles, plantar.
- Test balance, proprioception, fine motor movement.
- Test the cranial nerves if not previously tested.
- Test sensory perception.

GENITOURINARY SYSTEM

(Client standing and in lithotomy position)
- External and internal genitalia
- Pap smear
- Rectal examination
- Prostate examination

General Guidelines for Documentation of Findings

FREQUENCY

- Most acute care institutions require that a partial assessment be conducted and documented at the beginning of each shift. Other institutions require daily or weekly documentation of assessment findings (e.g., long-term care facilities and home health care agencies). A beginning-of-shift assessment could include:
  - Cardiovascular
  - Respiratory
  - Abdomen
  - Integumentary

- Musculoskeletal
- Gastrointestinal
- Urinary

SUGGESTIONS FOR EASE IN RECORDING

- Record findings on the form provided by the institution (if available).
- If the institution does not have a specific form for documenting assessment data, use the nurses' notes to record the assessment, following a systematic approach (based on a specific order of systems and a specific order within each system).
- Document (record) all normal and abnormal physical findings in a clear, organized, succinct, systematic manner.
- Use only professional abbreviations and terms accepted by the institution.
- Use a capital letter at the beginning and a period at the end of each statement. Use other punctuation as needed for clarity. Complete sentences are not necessary.
- Some institutions have bedside computer terminals so that assessment data can be recorded in the patient's room as soon as possible. Written data can usually be added to the hard copy.

PART 3

Body Organ and System Assessment

General Overview (With Examples)

Note and document the following information about the client:

- Apparent age (compared with stated or actual age)
- Weight (Note if clothing, shoes are included in measurements.)
- Height (remove the client's shoes)
- Arm span (equal to height except in older clients because of decreasing height with increasing age)
- Vital signs (Take BP in lying, sitting, and standing positions. Repeat in other arm if elevated.) Do not take BP in arm on mastectomy side or limb with dialysis access.
- Body type (tall, short, obese, thin, unusual body build)
- Posture (straight, stooped)
- Gait (fast, slow, limping, shuffling)
- Body movements (mannerisms, tremors)
- Obvious odors (alcohol, perfume, infection, poor hygiene)
- Personal hygiene (hair, oral hygiene, nails)
- Manner of dress (style, casual, hospital gown)
- Speech (clear, weak, slurred, hesitant, stuttering)
- Affect (flat, hostile, alert)
- Mood and manner (cheerful, depressed, crying)

Vital Signs

EQUIPMENT

- Thermometer, lubricant, watch with second hand, stethoscope, sphygmomanometer, gloves

ASSESSMENT OF THE ADULT

Health History

- Inquire about known temperature elevations, elevated blood pressure

  Temperature

- Secure appropriate thermometer, shake down to 96°F (35.5°C) if mercury-in-glass type.
- Oral: Place tip of thermometer near base of tongue, close lips. Keep in place 5 minutes if using mercury-in-glass thermometer or until beeps are completed if using electronic thermometer. Normal range is 97–100°F (36–37.8°C).
- Rectal: With client in left lateral Sims position, gently insert lubricated tip 1 to 1.5 inches. Hold in place 3 minutes if using mercury-in-glass thermometer or until beeps are completed if using electronic thermometer. Normal range is 98–101°F (37–38.8°C).
- Axillary: With client's arm raised, place tip of thermometer at center of axilla. Lower arm completely. Leave in place 7–10 minutes. Normal range is 96–99°F (35–36.8°C).

  Pulse

- Rate: Palpate radial pulse for 30 seconds and multiply times 2. Count for one full minute if irregular. Also assess for regular rhythm, strength (full, not bounding or thready), and equality (compare left and right). Normal range is 60–100 beats per minute.

Respiration

- Rate: Count breaths for 1 minute; normal range is 12–20 per minute. Also assess depth and rhythm and use of accessory muscles.

Blood Pressure

- Auscultate blood pressure in sitting position with brachial artery at level of heart. Auscultate in standing and lying positions. Reverse positions to assess postural hypotension. Repeat in other arm if elevated. Do not use the arm on the side of a mastectomy or dialysis access. Normal ranges:
  - Systolic 96–140 mm Hg
  - Diastolic 60–90 mm Hg

Integument

HISTORY

NOTE: A brief review of the essential components of the history is included at the beginning of each system. In many clinical situations the nurse will be concentrating primarily on one or more systems rather than a total integrated health assessment.

Adult

- Past skin diseases
- Years of exposure to sun and other environmental factors
- Recent change in a wart or mole
- Any sore that has not healed
- Rashes, lesions, abrasions, bruises
- Tick bites
- Adverse effects of medications
- Allergies, seasonal or climatic effects
- Recent changes in hair growth, distribution
- Recent changes in nails (e.g., ridges, thickening, color bands)

- Recent changes in sensation of pain, heat, cold
- Thyroid, endocrine, circulatory disorders

Pediatric

Infants

- Type of diaper and diaper cream used
- Method and products used for bath
- Rashes, lesions, bruises
- Injuries

Children

- Injury history related to play (e.g., abrasions, cuts)
- Signs of abuse
- Allergies
- Acne, eczema; include onset, treatment

Geriatric

- Past skin diseases
- Excessive dryness, itching
- Increased bruising tendency
- Increased healing time
- Chronic long-time sun exposure
- Marks (excoriation, redness, trauma)
- Temperature changes in skin
- Nail texture changes

EQUIPMENT

- 6″ transparent ruler measured in cm as well as inches
- Penlight or flashlight
- Gloves

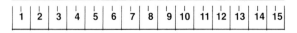

CENTIMETER SCALE

PATIENT PREPARATION

- Client sitting and standing for total exposure of skin
- Keep warm.
- Maintain complete privacy.

PHYSICAL ASSESSMENT—SKIN

Steps	Normal and/or Common Findings	Significant Deviations
Inspection		
• Color. Note symmetry, shade.	Pink, light brown, dark brown, ruddy, coffee, chloasma, vitiligo	Pale, cyanotic, jaundiced, sallow
• Lesions. Note size, location, shape, color.	Nevi, scars, keloids, especially in dark pigmented skin (see Fig. 2), striae	Tracks, varicosities, tick bites (whitened center with red circle around it)

Continued

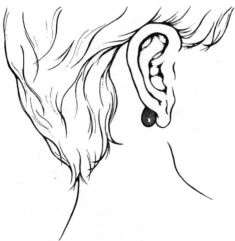

FIGURE 2.
Keloid lesion behind right ear.

Steps	Normal and/or Common Findings	Significant Deviations
• Erythema. Note location, size, blanching.	None	
• Lesions. Note type, morphology, location, size, shape, grouping or arrangement, exudate.	Macules	Papule, nodule, tumor, wheal, vesicle, bulla, pustule, erosion, excoriation, fissure, ulcer, scale, petechia, purpura, ecchymosis (see Table 2)

TABLE 2
TYPES OF SKIN LESIONS

Lesion	Size in cm	Description
Primary Lesions		
Macule	<1	Flat, circumscribed, varied in color
Papule	<1	Elevated, firm, solid
Nodule	1 < 2	Elevated, firm, solid
Tumor	>2	Elevated, firm, solid
Wheal	Varied	Transient, irregular, edematous
Vesicle	<1	Elevated, serous fluid–filled
Bulla	>1	Elevated, serous fluid–filled
Pustule	Varied	Elevated, purulent fluid–filled
Secondary Lesions		
Erosion	Varied	Moist epidermal depression; follows rupture of vesicle, bulla
Excoriation	Varied	Crusted epidermal abrasion
Fissure	Varied	Red, linear dermal break
Ulcer	Varied	Red dermal depression; exudate
Scale	Varied	Flaky, irregular, white to silver
Petechia	<0.5	Flat, red to purple
Purpura	>0.5	Flat, red to purple
Ecchymosis	Varied	Dark red to dark blue; painful

Steps	Normal and/or Common Findings	Significant Deviations
Smell		
• Odors	Cigarette smoke, perspiration	Alcohol, acetone, foul odors
Palpation		
• Temperature	Warm, cool	Hot, cold
• Turgor for degree (see Fig. 3)	Rebounds instantly	Tented for >5″
• Degree of moisture	Dry	Damp, clammy
• Texture	Smooth, even	Rough
• Lesions or lumps for pain, depth, size if not visible	None	Pain

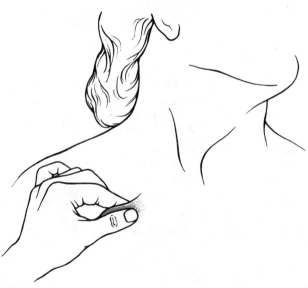

FIGURE 3.
Testing skin turgor.

PHYSICAL ASSESSMENT—HAIR

Steps	Normal and/or Common Findings	Significant Deviations
Inspection		
• Color	Black, brown, blond, red, gray, white	
• Quantity	Thick, thin	Patchy, none
• Distribution for presence, symmetry of body hair	Varies	Alopecia, marginal alopecia, hirsutism, absence on lower limbs
• General condition	Combed, clean	Dirty, uncombed, matted
Palpation		
• Texture	Coarse, fine, curly, oily, dry	Brittle

PHYSICAL ASSESSMENT—NAILS

Steps	Normal and/or Common Findings	Significant Deviations
Inspection		
• Plate for color	Pink, light brown	Blue, black
• Cuticle	Smooth	Edema, erythema, exudate
• Shape	Curved	Clubbed, flattened (see Fig. 21)
• Configuration (see Fig. 4)	Longitudinal ridges	Transverse depressions or ridges, pits
• General condition	Clean, neat	Unkept, dirty
Palpation		
• Consistency	Firm	Boggy, brittle

SPOON NAIL (KOILONYCHIA)

SPLINTER HEMORRHAGES

ONYCHOLYSIS

PARONYCHIA

TRANSVERSE GROOVING
(BEAU'S LINES)

FIGURE 4.
Abnormal nail conditions.

PEDIATRIC ADAPTATIONS

Infant

Steps	Normal and/or Common Findings	Significant Deviations
	SKIN	
Inspection		
• Color	Will usually reflect a lighter shade of parents' skin color at birth. Reddened to pink, acrocyanosis, mongolian spots, harlequin sign	Physiologic jaundice, nevus flammeus, cyanosis, purpura, multiple bruises, lesions that may be inconsistent with history

Continued

Steps	Normal and/or Common Findings	Significant Deviations
	SKIN (continued)	
• Texture	Smooth, soft. Vernix in creases, if term	
• Lesions	Milia	Capillary hemangioma, erythema toxicum
• Integrity	Intact	Openings, clefts especially on spine, head
• Palmar, sole creases for number, pattern	Multiple creases at term	Few to absent creases; simian line
Palpation		
• Turgor on abdomen	Instant recoil	Tenting
• Lesions for size, shape consistency		Café au lait spots >5 mm
	HAIR	
Inspection		
• General condition	Clean; cradle cap	
	NAILS	
Inspection		
• Size	Thin, may be long,	Clubbing
• Shape	easily cyanotic to	
• Color	pink	

Child

Steps	Normal and/or Common Findings	Significant Deviations
	SKIN	
Inspection		
• Color		Multiple bruises, burns

Steps	Normal and/or Common Findings	Significant Deviations
• Common diseases	Ringworm, impetigo, scabies	

HAIR		
Inspection		
• Foreign bodies	Color may darken and thicken	Head lice, nits, ticks

Adolescent

Steps	Normal and/or Common Findings	Significant Deviations
SKIN		
Inspection		
• Sebaceous glands	Oily, acne, comedones	

HAIR		
Inspection		
• Body hair. Note amount, pattern, texture.	Increases in amount, coarseness, progresses toward adult fullness and texture	Sparse, scanty, fine, patchy

GERIATRIC ADAPTATIONS

Steps	Normal and/or Common Findings	Significant Deviations
SKIN		
Inspection		
• Color	Lentigo senilis (back of hands, arms, face)	Erythema, bruises (head and trunk

Continued

Steps	Normal and/or Common Findings	Significant Deviations
	SKIN (continued)	
		more significant than arms or legs as possible signs of abuse)
• Temperature	Cool (lower temperature)	Uneven, asymmetrical, very cold
• Moisture	Dry, scaling, decreased perspiration	Cracked, fissured
• Texture	Thinning, transparent	
• Turgor (check on forehead, chest or abdomen) (see Fig. 3)	Wrinkling, decreased subcutaneous fat, sagging	Extended tenting
• Lesions (see Fig. 5)	Cherry angiomas, seborrheic keratosis, acrochordons, senile purpura	Actinic keratosis, basal cell carcinoma, squamous cell carcinoma
	HAIR	
Inspection		
• Color	Loss of pigment > age 50	
• Quantity	Decreased body hair, hirsutism, decreased hair on lower extremities, thinning of hair on head	Unusual alopecia, asymmetrical
	NAILS	
Inspection		
• Texture	Ridges, longitudinal splitting, thickening, decreased growth	

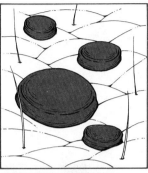

A, CHERRY ANGIOMA.

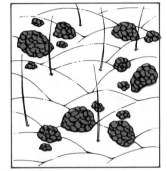

B, ACTINIC KERATOSIS.

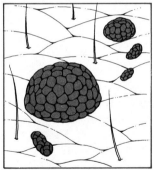

C, SEBORRHEIC KERATOSIS.

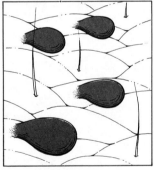

D, ACROCHORDON.

FIGURE 5.
Common skin changes in older adults. **A,** Cherry angioma. **B,** Actinic or senile keratosis. **C,** Seborrheic keratosis. **D,** Acrochordon.

DIAGNOSTIC TESTS

- Refer to physician for biopsy of suspicious lesions.

POSSIBLE NURSING DIAGNOSES

- Infection, high risk for
- Injury, high risk for
- Tissue integrity, impaired
- Skin integrity, impaired
- Skin integrity, impaired, high risk for
- Self-care deficit: Bathing/hygiene
- Body image disturbance
- Self-esteem disturbance

CLINICAL ALERT

- Refer all suspicious lesions.
- Report suspicious bruising.
- Note problems with cleanliness, grooming.

SAMPLE DOCUMENTATION

Skin bilaterally pale pink and elastic, with no varicosities, ecchymoses, edema, or erythema. Multiple striae present along lower abdomen and medial aspects of breasts. Abundant maculae scattered across nose, cheeks, and backs of ears. Raised white scar, 2 cm in diameter, on upper outer aspect of left arm. Skin on extremities symmetrical, cool, and dry. No noticeable odors. Hair thick, fine, light brown, and distributed normally on head. No hirsutism or hair loss noted. Nails slightly curved, firm, with no ridges or pits. Nail beds pink. No clubbing.

PATIENT/FAMILY EDUCATION AND HOME HEALTH NOTES

Adult

- Avoid exposure to sun as much as possible.
- Use sun screens >SPT 15 between 10 A.M. and 2 P.M. when

possible (dark and very dark skins may use a SPF as low as 4 to 6).

- Prevent clothing from irritating moles, warts, and other lesions.
- Do total self-assessment of skin monthly.
- Do not push cuticle back from nail surface.
- Inform client about special cosmetics for dark skin.

Pediatric

Infant

- Avoid sun exposure until 6 months of age, then use sunscreen.
- Teach parents about general and individual variations of normal.
- Instruct parents in cleansing and care of skin—mild soap, rinse well, oil only if very dry, no powders. Wash scalp and fontanels.
- Clip nails when infant is asleep or quiet.
- Change diapers frequently.
- When changing diapers, cleanse from pubis to anus.

Adolescent

- Wash with nondeodorant soap and water 2–3 × daily if skin is oily.

Geriatric

- Use soap sparingly and rinse well.
- Do not use alcohol or powder on skin.
- Bathing daily helps to retain moisture on skin.
- Use emollient lotion on chest, abdomen, back, arms, legs, and feet.
- Use emollient lotion after bathing on dry skin areas (avoid rubbing directly over pressure areas).
- Keep feet and between toes clean and dry.
- Use manicure stick rather than metal file to clean fingernails and toenails.

- Refer client to podiatrist if unable to safely trim and clean toenails.
- Prevent prolonged pressure to any area by position change, massage, and range of motion exercise.

Head

HISTORY

Adult

- Risk of head injury due to automobiles, cycling, sports, job, other
- Use of helmet and seatbelts
- History of head injury, seizures, headaches
- Headache: location, onset, duration, character of pain, precipitating factors, treatment
- Stress management techniques

Pediatric

- Birth trauma, difficult delivery
- Neural tube defects
- Injuries (trauma)

Geriatric

- Syncope, headaches, trauma

EQUIPMENT

- Tape measure
- Pin or cotton ball
- Flashlight or penlight
- Stethoscope

PATIENT PREPARATION

- Sitting

PHYSICAL ASSESSMENT

Steps	Normal and/or Common Findings	Significant Deviations
Inspection		
• Head. Note position, movements, facial features, symmetry, shape, expressions.	Upright Still	Tilted to one side, involuntary movements Tremor, bobbing, nodding Tics, spasms
	Slight asymmetry	Asymmetry (entire side, partial, mouth only)
	Uniform	Edema, unusual shapes
	Appropriate	Flat, fixed
Palpation		
• Skull. Note shape, symmetry.	Smooth, uniform, intact	Lump, indentations
• Temporal arteries. Note course.	Smooth, nontender	Tenderness, thickening
• Temporomandibular joint. Note range of motion.	3–6 cm vertical range when mouth open; 1–2 cm lateral motion; snaps or pops	Pain Crepitus Inability to close or open fully
Test		
• Cranial nerve (CN) VII: Have client puff cheeks, raise brows, frown, smile.	Symmetrical movement	Asymmetrical motion or absence of motion
• CN V: Have client clench teeth. Touch pin or cotton ball to chin, cheek, forehead.	Symmetrical movement Symmetrical response	Asymmetrical motion or absence of motion Asymmetrical or absent perception of touch

Continued

Steps	Normal and/or Common Findings	Significant Deviations
Auscultation (Only if vascular anomaly suspected; use bell only)		
• Temples, eyes, suboccipital areas		Bruits

PEDIATRIC ADAPTATIONS

Infants

Steps	Normal and/or Common Findings	Significant Deviations
Inspection		
• Skull. Note size, shape, symmetry (see Fig. 6).	Molding Caput succedaneum, flat fontanels, long narrow shape if premature	Cephalohematoma, Dilated scalp veins
Palpation		
• Fontanels. Note size, tension, suture lines.	<5 cm anterior, slight pulsation, soft fontanel	Marked pulsations or depressed fontanels; bulging, full fontanels Nonpalpable sutures Extra ridges, craniotabes
Measure		
• Occipital frontal circumference	Should approximate chest circumference	Micro/macrocephaly
Transilluminate (Only if abnormality is suspected)	Light does not penetrate skull.	Light glows through cranial cavity

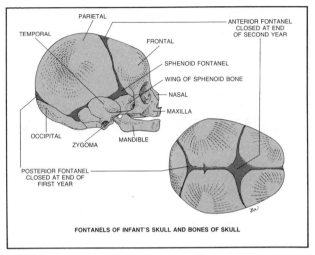

FIGURE 6.
Fontanels of infant's skull and bones of skull. (Source: Taber's, 17th ed., p 747 with permission.)

CHILDREN

Steps	Normal and/or Common Findings	Significant Deviations
Auscultation		
• Eyes, temples, sub-occiput	Bruits common until age 5	Bruits after age 5

GERIATRIC ADAPTATIONS

None

DIAGNOSTIC TESTS

May need to refer for:
- CT scan
- MRI

POSSIBLE NURSING DIAGNOSES

- Trauma, high risk for
- Tissue perfusion, altered: cerebral
- Injury, high risk for
- Body image disturbance

CLINICAL ALERT

- Pediatric
  - Cephalohematoma
  - Bulging or depressed fontanels
  - Microcephaly
  - Macrocephaly
- Adult, Geriatric
  - Bruits
  - Asymmetry if marked or new
  - Hardness, thickening, or tenderness over temporal arteries may be associated with temporal arteritis.
  - Enlarged occipital, preauricular/postauricular lymph nodes

SAMPLE DOCUMENTATION

Face symmetrical without involuntary movements. CN V, VII intact. Skull smooth, symmetrical. Expressions appropriate to setting.

PATIENT/FAMILY EDUCATION AND HOME HEALTH NOTES

Adult

- Always use helmet when cycling
- Always use seat belts
- Basic stress management techniques

Pediatric

- Explain various skull shapes due to birth and indicate expected recovery time.

- Explain fontanels, including that they can be touched, and that hair should be washed.
- Strongly encourage use of helmets when riding bicycles or skateboarding; use of car seats, seat belts (mandatory in most states).

Geriatric

- Safety tips related to dizziness
- Avoid falls. Do not use throw rugs, use safety grips on floor of bathtub, label stairs well, use night light in bathroom.
- Rise from lying to standing position slowly if dizziness occurs
- Use cane or walker if indicated.

Neck

HISTORY

Adult

- Recent weight changes
- Changes in activity tolerance; fatigue, irritability
- Thyroid disease or surgery
- Neck stiffness or pain
- Temperature intolerance
- Difficulty swallowing
- Enlarged lymph nodes
- Radiation exposure
- Chemotherapy
- HIV exposure
- IV drug use
- Recurrent infections
- Hoarseness

Pediatric

Infant

- Maternal hyperthyroidism

Geriatric

- Thyroid disease, especially hypothyroidism
- Stiff neck muscles

EQUIPMENT

- Stethoscope

PATIENT PREPARATION

- Sitting
- May need cup of water for client to swallow during thyroid palpation

PHYSICAL ASSESSMENT

Steps	Normal and/or Common Findings	Significant Deviations
Inspection		
• Neck. Note shape, symmetry, size.	Uniform, symmetrical, proportional to head and shoulders	Masses, webbing or fullness Unusually short Edema
• Trachea. Note position.	Midline	Deviations to either side
• Carotid, jugular	Mild pulsations	Distention, fullness
• Thyroid (with and without swallowing). Note symmetry, size.	Usually not visible	Marked
Palpation		
• Trachea. Note position, margins, motion (finger and thumb held on either side of trachea; feel for downward pull that is synchronous with pulse).	Midline, nontender, distinct rings	Edematous, deviated laterally, tender or painful, tracheal tugging

Steps	Normal and/or Common Findings	Significant Deviations
• Thyroid. Note size, shape consistency, tenderness: place two fingers on each side of trachea below cricoid cartilage. Feel for isthmus while client swallows. Gently push trachea to right side, have client tilt head to left side, feel right lobe while client swallows. Reverse and repeat. Palpate lateral borders by pressing on either side of each sternocleidomastoid as client swallows (Fig. 7)	May be nonpalpable. Right lobe may be slightly larger if palpable with swallowing.	Enlarged, tender, nodules, masses, roughened surface Fixed
• Lymph nodes. Note location, mobility, size, shape, consistency, tenderness, skin margins, color. (Begin with light pressure, gradually increasing to moderate pressure.) See Fig. 8 for nodes to palpate.	Nonpalpable; small ($\leq$1 cm), smooth firm, mobile, nontender, discrete margins	Inflamed nodes: enlarged, tender, mobile, blurred borders, reddened skin Malignant nodes: enlarged, nontender, fixed, hard, nodular, irregular shape, nondiscrete margins
Testing		
• CN XI. Have client shrug shoulders with and without resistance, and	Symmetrical movement and strength	Asymmetrical or absent motion

Continued

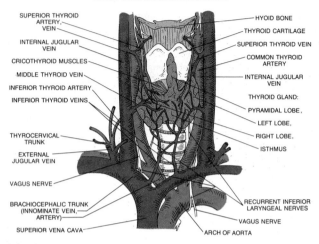

FIGURE 7.
Thyroid gland and related structures. (Source: Taber's, 17th ed., p 1995 with permission.)

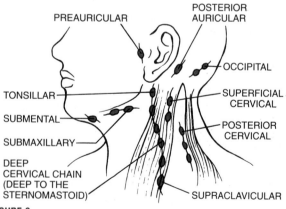

FIGURE 8.
Lymph nodes of the head and neck.

Steps	Normal and/or Common Findings	Significant Deviations
have client turn head to each side against resistance.		
Auscultation		
• Enlarged thyroid. Note bruits (use bell).	None	Bruits
• Carotid arteries. Note bruit.	None	Bruits (e.g., from aortic stenosis)

PEDIATRIC ADAPTATIONS

Steps	Normal and/or Common Findings	Significant Deviations
Inspection		
• Assess ROM of neck. Note nuchal rigidity, if any.	Full ROM	Webbing Nuchal rigidity Edema
Palpation		
• Thyroid	May be palpable, nontender Lymph nodes may be palpable	
• <2 yr: postauricular and occipital; > 1 yr: cervical, submandibular		

GERIATRIC ADAPTATIONS

Steps	Normal and/or Common Findings	Significant Deviations
Inspection		
• ROM. Note flexibility, strength.	Decreased	Stiff

Continued

Steps	Normal and/or Common Findings	Significant Deviations
Palpation		
• Thyroid	Irregular surface, fibrous changes	
• Lymph nodes	May be fibrous	

DIAGNOSTIC TESTS

May need to refer for:
- Infant screen: hypothyroidism
- Biopsy of enlarged lymph nodes
- Thyroid-stimulating hormone (TSH), triiodothyronine (T_3), thyroxin (T_4), (T_7)

POSSIBLE NURSING DIAGNOSES

- Airway clearance, ineffective
- Activity intolerance, high risk for
- Swallowing, impaired
- Aspiration, high risk for

CLINICAL ALERT

- Obstructed airway
- Palpable supraclavicular nodes always referred
- Refer any suspicious nodes
- Refer enlarged, nodular thyroid
- Hypothyroidism frequently not diagnosed in older clients and assumed to be depression

SAMPLE DOCUMENTATION

Neck smooth, supple, with full ROM. Trachea aligned in midline. Neither jugular nor carotid distended. Thyroid not visible, not palpable. No tenderness. CN XI intact. Lymph nodes (auricular, occipital, clavicular, cervical, tonsillar, submaxillary, submental) not palpable.

PATIENT/FAMILY EDUCATION AND HOME HEALTH NOTES

Adult

- Self-referral of enlarged suspicious nodes, difficulty swallowing

Pediatric

- Infants—thoroughly clean skin folds in neck.
- Infants—no pillows or soft stuffed animals should be allowed in crib.
- Never shake infant or child (significant risk for injury to head or neck).

Geriatric

- Thyroid tests if patient reports low energy
- Exercise neck muscles to maintain as much mobility as possible (flexion, extension, hyperextension, rotation, lateral flexion).
- If several pillows are used, place part of pillows under shoulder to prevent prolonged extreme neck flexion.

Eyes

HISTORY

Adult

- Date and source of last eye exam; age at time of exam
- Use of corrective lenses; if so, type, how long
- History (self or family) of hypertension, diabetes, allergies, thyroid disorder, glaucoma, medications
- History of prior eye surgery, trauma, infection

- Headache
- Pain, burning, itching, drying, tearing, discharge
- Blurred vision
- Lights, spots, floaters
- Recent changes in vision

Pediatric

- Maternal rubella while pregnant
- Ability to follow object and fixate with eyes
- Squinting to see objects; rubbing of eyes
- Age, Date and source of last eye exam; age at time of exam
- Headaches when reading
- Reversals of written numbers and/or letters
- Trouble reading correctly
- Does child sit close to the television at home?

Geriatric

- Increased difficulty reading, seeing at night; peripheral or central vision blurred
- Blood relative who had glaucoma
- Long, excessive exposure to sunlight
- Bothered by glaring lights
- Bothered by rainbows around lights

EQUIPMENT

- Penlight
- Rosenbaum chart or newsprint
- Snellen chart
- Ophthalmoscope
- Clean cotton wisp
- Cover card

PATIENT PREPARATION

- Sitting position
- Explain darkening of room for ophthalmic exam.
- Explain use of cotton to elicit blink.

PHYSICAL ASSESSMENT—EXTERNAL EYES

Steps	Normal and/or Common Findings	Significant Deviations
Inspection		
• Bony orbit, brows, lacrimal apparatus, eye. Note symmetry, size, position (Fig. 9).	Equal size and movement	Exophthalmos Strabismus
• Lids. Note position, motion, symmetry, lesions.	Symmetrical blink, lashes even and curl out, moist Xanthelasma	Edema, ptosis, exudate, ectropion, hordeolum
• Iris. Note color, shape.	Uniform color, round	Coloboma, iridectomy
• Cornea, lens (with oblique light)	Clear, smooth, moist	Opaque, arcus senilis before age 40
• Pupil. Note shape, symmetry, response to light	PERRLA Consensual	Not equal in shape, response to light unequal, slow, absent, diminished
• Note cloudiness of lens		Cataract
• Pupil. Note accommodation—focus distant object, then close (Fig. 10)	Constricts for close object	Miosis, mydriasis Fails to respond to focus change

Continued

NORMAL EYES

EPICANTHAL FOLDS

WIDE-SET EYES

PALPEBRAL SLANT

FIGURE 9.
Placement of the eyes.

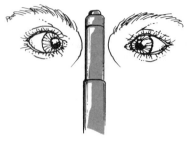

FIGURE 10.
Checking for accommodation.

Steps	Normal and/or Common Findings	Significant Deviations
• Conjunctiva. Note color, continuity, vascularity	Clear with multiple small vessels	Reddened, exudate, lesions, jaundice
Palpation		
• Bony orbit	Firm, nontender	Tenderness
• Lacrimal apparatus	Pink, moist puncta	Tenderness, drainage, reddened, edema
Testing Eye Function		
• CN II. Rosenbaum chart at 14 in (Fig. 11) Have client cover one eye; test uncovered eye. Test with lenses if client already uses glasses of contacts. Test OD, OS, OU.	20/20 without straining Near vision: reads at 14 in	Decreased acuity, e.g., 20/40 Moves closer or further than 14 in for reading

Continued

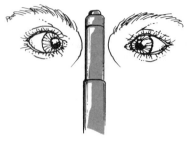

FIGURE 11.
Rosenbaum pocket vision screener. (Source: Dr. J. George Rosenbaum, F.A.C.S., Cleveland, Ohio, with permission.)

ROSENBAUM POCKET VISION SCREENER

Card is held in good light 14 inches from eye. Record vision for each eye separately with and without glasses. Presbyopic patients should read thru bifocal segment. Check myopes with glasses only.

					Point	Jaeger	Distance Equivalent
95							$\frac{20}{800}$
874							$\frac{20}{400}$
2843					26	16	$\frac{20}{200}$
638	ᗐШᗐ		XOO		14	10	$\frac{20}{100}$
8745	ᗐШШ		OXO		10	7	$\frac{20}{70}$
63925	Шᗐᗐᗐᗐ		XOX		8	5	$\frac{20}{50}$
428365	ШᗐШ		o x o		6	3	$\frac{20}{40}$
374258	ᗐШᗐ		X X O		5	2	$\frac{20}{30}$
937826	ШᗐШ		x o o		4	1	$\frac{20}{25}$
428739	ᗐШШ		o o x		3	1+	$\frac{20}{20}$

PUPIL GAUGE (mm.)

2 3 4 5 6 7 8 9

Steps	Normal and/or Common Findings	Significant Deviations
• Confrontation test. With your eyes level with client's eyes, stand 2 ft from client and cover one eye while client covers opposite eye. Look at each other. Move object into superior, inferior, nasal, and temporal fields for each eye (Fig. 12).	Object is seen by both at same time	Diminished peripheral vision
• CN III, IV, VI and extraocular muscles. Hold client's chin, have client focus eyes on pencil held at comfortable distance from eyes; instruct client to follow pencil with eyes as pencil is moved through six cardinal fields of gaze (Fig. 13).	Smooth, equal movements	Nystagmus Lid lag
• Shine light obliquely into each pupil.	Equal pupillary constriction	Asymmetry or absence of pupillary constriction
• Muscle balance with corneal light reflex. Shine light on corneas while client looks straight ahead.	Symmetrical reflection of light	Asymmetry: strabismus, hypertelorism
• CN V. Touch wisp of cotton to cornea to elicit blink reflex (alert client before touching with cotton).	Blink symmetrical and complete	Asymmetrical, incomplete, or absent blink response

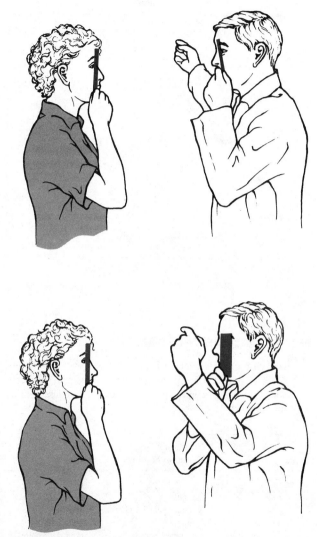

FIGURE 12.
Testing peripheral fields of vision.

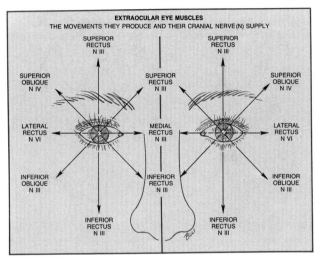

FIGURE 13.
Extraocular eye muscles. (Source: Taber's, 17th ed., p 696 with permission.)

PHYSICAL ASSESSMENT—INTERNAL EYES

- Darken room. Have client focus on object over your shoulder. OD: ophthalmoscope in right hand, focus with numbered wheel. OS: ophthalmoscope in left hand. (Procedure is tiring for client.)

Steps	Normal and/or Common Findings	Significant Deviations
Inspection		
• Red reflex	Present	Cataract, hemorrhage
	Round, reddish-orange	may appear solid or as dots.
• Retina. Note color.	Yellowish pink, uniform	Marked dark colors, lesions, folds in retina

Steps	Normal and/or Common Findings	Significant Deviations
• Disc. Note color, size, shape, margins of disc and cup.	Yellow to pink, round, 1.5 mm, sharply defined border, cup 40–50% of disc, lighter color in center of disc	Papilledema, cupping with white color, vessels visible in disc Cup less or more than 40–50% of disc
• Vessels. Note color, size, junctions	Size A3:V5, arterioles bright red	AV nicking, areas of constriction
• Macula densa and fovea centralis. Note location, color (Fig. 14) (difficult to locate unless pupils are dilated).	Located two disc diameters temporal to disk, bright yellow	

PEDIATRIC ADAPTATIONS

Infant

Steps	Normal and/or Common Findings	Significant Deviations
Inspection		
• External eye. Note spacing, symmetry.	Symmetrically positioned and spaced	Edema of lids, epicanthal folds (abnormal except in Asians), hypertelorism
• Ability of infant to gaze at parent and blink appropriately (see Fig. 9)		Failure to gaze and blink
• Conjunctiva. Note color, clarity.	Pink, moist	Drainage

Continued

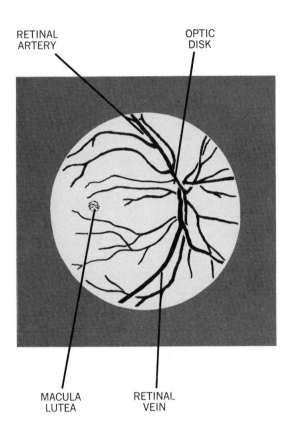

RETINA OF RIGHT EYE

FIGURE 14.
Retina of right eye. (Source: Taber's 17th ed., p. 1709 with permission.)

Steps	Normal and/or Common Findings	Significant Deviations
• Muscle balance	Symmetrical movement, pseudostrabismus	Strabismus, nystagmus
• Red reflex	Present	
Child Testing		
• Visual acuity (Snellen symbol chart for ages 3–7; not accurate < age 3)	Age 1: 20/200 Age 2: 20/70 Age 5: 20/30 Age 6: 20/20	
• Color differentiation check at age 5	Differentiates colors	Color blindness

GERIATRIC ADAPTATIONS

Steps	Normal and/or Common Findings	Significant Deviations
Inspection		
• Lids. Note position.		Lid lag, ptosis, ectropion, entropion
• Pupils. Note size	Diminished	
• Cornea. Note clarity.	Arcus senilis Diminished visual acuity Diminished adaptation to dark	
• Lens. Note clarity.	Clear	Cloudiness, opacity

PHYSICAL ASSESSMENT—INTERNAL EYES

- Darken room. Have client focus on object over your shoulder. OD: ophthalmoscope in right hand, focus with numbered wheel. OS: ophthalmoscope in left hand. (Procedure is tiring for client.)

DIAGNOSTIC TESTS

May need to refer for:
- Mydriatic agent—to dilate pupils for full fundoscopic exam
- Puff test for pressure in glaucoma

POSSIBLE NURSING DIAGNOSES

- Sensory-perceptual alterations: Visual
- Social interaction, impaired
- Social isolation

CLINICAL ALERT

- Explain possible discomfort of light and cotton wisp.
- Do not use light in eyes for excessively long times.
- If red reflex is absent, reposition scope.

SAMPLE DOCUMENTATION

Eyes: Symmetrical with no lag or turning of lids; no exoph-thalmos noted. Sclera clear, white; conjunctiva dark pink without inflammation. Irises light blue, intact. PERRLA. EOMs and normal visual fields intact (CN III, IV, VI). Alignment and convergence normal. Corneal reflex intact (CN V). Fundoscopic: discs flat, yellow. No AV nicking, hemorrhage, or cupping noted; A3:V5. Acuity (CN II): OD 20/40, OS 20/20, OU 20/20. Corrected (Rosenbaum chart).

PATIENT/FAMILY EDUCATION AND HOME HEALTH NOTES

Adult

- Examination every 5 to 10 years until age 40, then every 2 to 5 years
- Use of safety glasses with hobbies, home repair

Pediatric

Infants

- Explain normal vision; i.e., poor acuity and poor muscle control at birth, lack of tears until 3 months.

Children and Adolescents

- Use sunglasses when outdoors, especially when in the sun or in highly reflective areas (for example, sand, water, snow).
- Vision screening at ages 3, 4 to 6, 7 to 9, and 13 years of age
- Color screening at 4 to 5 years of age

Geriatric

- Explain drying of mucous membranes, possible need for artificial lubricants.
- Recommend examination every year and as necessary when changes occur.
- Emphasize that blindness due to glaucoma or cataracts is preventable or treatable if detected early and that eye drops for glaucoma must be taken for a lifetime.
- Inform client of visual side effects of any medications being taken.

Ears

HISTORY

Adult

- Changes in hearing acuity
- Aids to hearing used
- Vertigo, earaches, drainage
- Exposure to loud sounds
- Medications affecting hearing, especially antibiotics
- Methods of hygiene

- History of renal disease, diabetes
- History of sinusitis, streptococcal infections
- History of Ménière's disease
- History of ear surgery, trauma

Pediatric

- Maternal syphilis, rubella
- Exposure to antibiotics
- Chronic otitis media or upper respiratory infections
- Exposure to passive smoke
- Pulling or tugging ears
- No increasing pattern of speech-babbling, speech
- Foul odor

Adolescents

- Exposure to loud noises—chronic, acute, amount
- Frequency and sites of swimming
- Protrusion of external ear

Geriatric

- Ringing or cracking noises
- Do conversations of others sound garbled or distorted?
- If hearing aid is used, is it effective?

EQUIPMENT

- Otoscope
- Tuning fork
- Ticking watch

PATIENT PREPARATION

- Client sitting
- Tip head away from ear being examined
- Parent may hold infant or toddler against parent's chest for otoscope exam

PHYSICAL ASSESSMENT—EXTERNAL EAR

Steps	Normal and/or Common Findings	Significant Deviations
Inspection		
• Position of ear in relation to eye (Fig. 15)	Ear should be nearly upright, angling < 10° toward occiput.	Unequal alignment, pinna below line level with corner of eye
• Auricles. Note size, shape, color, symmetry.	Color of skin, uniform shape	Masses, lesions, deformities, cyanosis erythema, edema
Palpation		
• Ear lobes	Smooth, uniform edge	Tophi, nodules

Continued

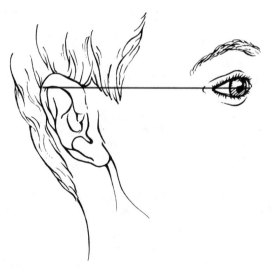

FIGURE 15.
Position of eye and ear.

Steps	Normal and/or Common Findings	Significant Deviations
• Tragus, helix	Nontender	Tenderness, pain, ulcers
• Mastoid	Nontender	Edema, tenderness, masses

Testing Hearing Function

Test CN VIII

• Weber. Place vibrating fork at midsagittal line (Fig. 16).	Client should hear or sense vibrations equally in both ears.	Sound lateralized to one ear: Perceptive loss due to nerve damage—goes to unaffected ear. Conductive loss due to otosclerosis—goes to affected ear.
• Rinne. Place vibrating fork on mastoid: after vibrations are no longer felt, hold beside ear to hear (Fig. 16).	Air conduction = 2 × bone conduction; able to hear vibrations after feeling stops (air conduction greater than bone conduction).	If air conduction >2 × bone conduction, there is perceptive loss. If air conduction <2 × bone conduction, there is conductive loss
• CN VIII. Occlude one of client's ears and whisper 1–2 ft lateral to opposite ear.	Client should be able to hear half of all words whispered.	Unable to hear
• Watch test. Start at about 18 in away from ear and compare with a person with normal hearing.	Able to hear at approximately the same distance as others with normal hearing heard the same watch.	Unable to hear

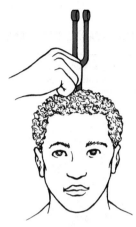

WEBER TEST

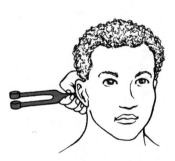
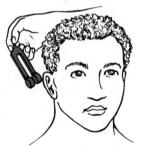

RINNE TEST

FIGURE 16.
Weber test and Rinne test.

PHYSICAL ASSESSMENT—CANAL, MEMBRANE

Steps	Normal and/or Common Findings	Significant Deviations
Inspection		
Anchor otoscope on client's head, tilted away from you; pull auricle up, out, and back to straighten auditory canal and *gently* insert speculum to depth of approximately ½ in (Fig. 17).		
• Canal. Note appearance of canal color; amount, type, and site of cerumen.	Moist cerumen, cilia	Foreign bodies, discharge, lesions, foul odor, edema, flaking, erythema, moderate to severe pain on insertion Completely occluded canal
• Tympanic membrane. Note landmarks (umbo, cone of light, malleus handles) color (Fig. 18), integrity.	Silver-gray color, shiny, conical, intact. Old scars appear as white marks. Cone of light at 5 o'clock position in right ear and at 7 o'clock position in left ear.	Bulging (unable to note landmarks) or retracting (pronounced landmarks) Perforations, foul odor, discharge Dull, red, blue

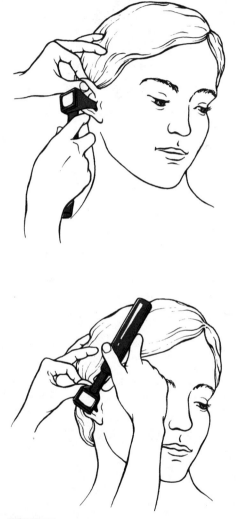

FIGURE 17.
Use of otoscope.

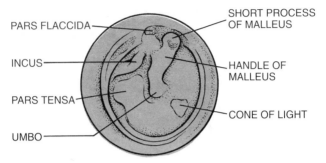

PARS FLACCIDA

INCUS

PARS TENSA

UMBO

SHORT PROCESS OF MALLEUS

HANDLE OF MALLEUS

CONE OF LIGHT

FIGURE 18.
The tympanic membrane and landmarks.

PEDIATRIC ADAPTATIONS

Infant

Steps	Normal and/or Common Findings	Significant Deviations
Inspection		
• External. Note shape and placement. Draw an imaginary line from the inner canthus of the eye to the outer canthus of the eye.	Uniform size and shape Recoils briskly Top of ear intersects this line	Preauricular pits, dimples, skin tags Unusual shapes Low-set ears Slow or absent recoil Foul odor
• Canal. Stabilize head, restrain child firmly if needed, gently pull auricle down and back.	Vernix in canal	
• Tympanic membrane. Use pneumatic otoscope to	If membrane is red, may be due to crying. Flattened	Fluid, edema, bulging, marked reddening

Steps	Normal and/or Common Findings	Significant Deviations
differentiate from illness.		Loss of bony landmarks Nonmobile tympanic membrane
Test		
• Infant	Startle (Moro) or blink reflex	Delayed or absent response
• 4–6 months old	Turns to sounds	
• 8–10 months old	Responds to name	
• 12 months old	Begins to imitate words	
• 3–4 years old Use Weber or Rinne test		

GERIATRIC ADAPTATIONS

Steps	Normal and/or Common Findings	Significant Deviations
Inspection		
• Auricles. Note size.		Women may have large sagging lobes if they have worn heavy earrings for many years.
• Cerumen. Note amount and consistency.		Dry, black, impacted cerumen

DIAGNOSTIC TESTS

May need to refer for:
• Audiometric testing

POSSIBLE NURSING DIAGNOSES

- Communication, impaired verbal
- Social isolation
- Self-esteem disturbance
- Injury, high risk for

CLINICAL ALERT

- Refer to otolaryngologist for severe tenderness, pain, lesions, discharge, foreign bodies, and/or progressive hearing loss

SAMPLE DOCUMENTATION

Verbal and nonverbal communication congruent and appropriate to setting. Ears aligned well on head. Pinnae pink, elastic, symmetrical, without lesions, deformities, or tenderness. Moderate amount of dark brown moist cerumen in canal; no lesions or redness. Tympanic membrane, shiny, gray, visible in both ears. Landmarks noted; no bulges, retractions, or redness. Vibratory sense intact. CN VIII intact with whisper test.

PATIENT/FAMILY EDUCATION AND HOME HEALTH NOTES

Adult

- Do not attempt to clean or remove wax with a cotton swab or other device.
- Use washcloth or finger in outer ear.
- If canal needs cleaning, irrigate with bulb syringe, soaking with oil if necessary.
- Avoid excessively loud sounds or use ear plugs.

Pediatric

- Ear infections are common and potentially dangerous. Do not put to bed with bottles of milk or other fluids. Be aware that colds and mild upper respiratory infections may develop into ear infections.

- Explain increased risk of otitis media for infants through preschoolers.
- Clean only outer ear using damp cloth.
- Child may insert objects into ears. Take child to health care provider for removal of all objects.
- Audiometric testing should be given to preschooler.

Geriatric

- Have hearing tested annually by a physician or audiologist.
- Obtain a variety of hearing devices for the home, such as louder bells on telephone and door chimes.
- Teach about hearing aids and how to care for them, and to purchase one only if recommended by a physician or audiologist. Purchase from a reputable company.

Nose and Sinuses

HISTORY

Adult

- Stuffiness; discharge (character, onset, duration, treatment)
- Sore throat
- Infections
- Epistaxis (cause, duration, treatment)
- Allergies; use of nose drops/sprays
- Repeated sinus infections
- Changes in appetite, smell sense
- Cocaine use
- History of surgery/trauma

Pediatric

- Nasal quality to voice
- "Allergic salute"
- Rhinitis

Geriatric

- Constant drip from nose to throat
- Allergies, sneezing
- Pain

EQUIPMENT

- Penlight
- Nasal speculum

PATIENT PREPARATION

- Sitting

PHYSICAL ASSESSMENT—EXTERNAL

Steps	Normal and/or Common Findings	Significant Deviations
Inspection		
• Nose. Note shape, symmetry, color discharge.	Varies Uniform, symmetrical, scant	Bullous, flaring, discharge (watery, purulent, mucoid, bloody) mucus, crusting
Palpation		
• Nose. Note masses, tenderness.	Straight, nontender	Masses, tenderness
• Patency. With client's mouth closed, occlude each naris to assess patency of opposite side.	Patent	Occluded
• Frontal sinuses. Press upward with thumbs under brow ridge.	Nontender	Tenderness, pain

Steps	Normal and/or Common Findings	Significant Deviations
• Maxillary sinuses. Press up with thumbs under zygomatic arch, press in over maxillary sinus.	Nontender	Tenderness, pain
Test		
• CN I. Test each naris separately for ability to perceive and identify odors. Use a different scent for each naris.	Distinguishes odors	Unable to distinguish odors
Percussion		
• Frontal and maxillary sinuses	Nontender	Tenderness, edema

PHYSICAL ASSESSMENT—INTERNAL

Steps	Normal and/or Common Findings	Significant Deviations
Inspection		
Tilt head back to insert speculum 1 cm. Avoid touching septum with speculum.		
• Nares. Note color, mucosa	Pink and moist	Masses, lesions, redness, foreign bodies Polyps, fissures, ulcers, discharge, bleeding

Continued

Steps	Normal and/or Common Findings	Significant Deviations
• Inferior, middle, and superior turbiantes. Note color, consistency.	Pink, smooth (same color as mucosa)	Redness, pallor, edema
• Septum. Note integrity, alignment.	Straight Uniform	Deviation due to trauma, bleeding

PEDIATRIC ADAPTATIONS

Infant

Steps	Normal and/or Common Findings	Significant Deviations
Inspection		
• Nose. Note shape of bridge.	Straight	

Child

Steps	Normal and/or Common Findings	Significant Deviations
Inspection		
• Nose. Note horizontal crease. Note if mouth or nose breather.	No crease Breathes through nose	"Allergic salute" possible sign of allergies Consistently breathes through mouth; clearly audible breath sounds
• Sphenoid, maxillary, ethmoid sinus (preschool child)	Nontender	Tender
• Frontal sinus (7–8 years of age)	Nontender	Tender

GERIATRIC ADAPTATIONS

Steps	Normal and/or Common Findings	Significant Deviations
Inspection		
• Nose. Note size.	Becomes larger and more prominent with age	
Test		
• Sense of smell	Diminishes with age	Absent

DIAGNOSTIC TESTS

May need to refer for:
• Biopsy of suspicious lesions

POSSIBLE NURSING DIAGNOSES

- Breathing pattern, ineffective
- Injury, high risk for
- Airway clearance, ineffective
- Aspiration, high risk for
- Communication, impaired verbal

CLINICAL ALERT

• Prevent trauma to nasal mucosa with use of nasal speculum, nasal catheter, or nasogastric feeding tube.

SAMPLE DOCUMENTATION

Nose aligned, symmetrical, without discharge or redness. Both nares patent, no tenderness or masses palpated. Mucosa and septum without redness, swelling, or lesions. Sinuses not tender. CN I intact; distinguishes smells independently.

PATIENT/FAMILY EDUCATION AND HOME HEALTH NOTES

Adult

- Prevent trauma to sensitive mucous membranes of nose.

Pediatric

- Avoid insertion of foreign bodies into nose. If object has been inserted, take child to physician's office for removal if foreign body is not easily grasped.
- Demonstrate use of tissue and handwashing to prevent spread of upper respiratory infection (URI).

Geriatric

- If sense of smell is diminished, teach client to routinely check and turn off dials on gas stoves (to prevent asphyxiation) and to label with a specific date foods stored in the refrigerator (to prevent eating spoiled foods).
- Inspect pilot lights periodically to lessen risk of gas exposure.
- Have smoke detector installed in home and test every 6 months.

Mouth and Throat

HISTORY

Adult

- Oral hygiene practices (method, frequency)
- Nutritional habits
- Tobacco use (type, frequency, duration)
- Alcohol use (frequency, duration)
- Pain
- Lesions
- Sore throat
- Hoarseness, change in voice
- Cough
- Difficulty chewing or swallowing
- History of herpes simplex, diabetes mellitus, periodontal disease

Pediatric

- Dental hygiene
- Number of teeth present
- Fluoridated water
- Use of bottle/pacifier
- Thumb sucking
- Sore throats

Geriatric

- Date of last dental examination
- Alterations in taste
- If prosthetic devices are used, note wearing habits and difficulties.

EQUIPMENT

- Light
- Gloves (clean)
- Gauze square
- Tongue depressor

PATIENT PREPARATION

- Sitting

PHYSICAL ASSESSMENT

Steps	Normal and/or Common Findings	Significant Deviations
Inspection		
• Lips. Note color, symmetry, continuity at squamous/ buccal junction (Fig. 19).	Pink, slight asymmetry, intact	Lesions, involuntary movement, cracks, fissures, drooping, cyanosis
• Mucosa and gums. Note color, integrity, adherence.	Pink, intact, moist	Redness, edema, lesions, masses, bleeding, cyanosis

Continued

MOUTH, TONGUE, AND PHARYNX

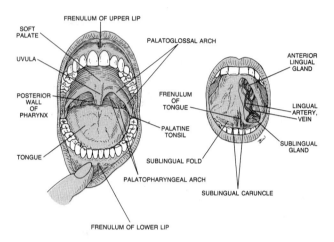

FIGURE 19.
Mouth, tongue, and pharynx. (Source: Taber's, 17th ed., p 1242 with permission.)

Steps	Normal and/or Common Findings	Significant Deviations
• Stenson's and Wharton's ducts. Note color.	Smooth, pink	Redness, edema
• Teeth. Note number, color, hygiene.	Complete, white, clean	Multiple caries, missing teeth, fuzzy, dirty
• Tongue. Note size. Check lateral, dorsal, and ventral surfaces for color, coating, texture, vessels.	Fits comfortably in mouth with teeth together Pink to red with papillae present Midline fissures present Geographic tongue	Coated, white patches, pale, nodules, ulcers Papillae or fissures absent

Steps	Normal and/or Common Findings	Significant Deviations
• Palate, oropharynx, uvula. Note color, continuity, integrity	Pink. Hard palate firm with rugae, soft palate spongy, uvula in midline	Redness, edema, lesions Uvula deviated (Note direction) Softened hard palate
• Tonsils. Note color, size, discharge.	Pink to red 1+ to 2+	Exudate 3+ to 4+ Markedly reddened

Test

| • CN XII. Have client extend tongue and move side to side. | Tongue should centrally align without fasciculations. | No central alignment, fasciculations |
| • CN IX, X. Observe soft palate and uvula rising as client says "ah"; after alerting client, gently touch back of tongue with tongue depressor to elicit gag reflex. | Soft palate rises symmetrically, uvula in midline, quick gag reflex | Unequal or absent rise of soft palate, uvula deviated on rising
Absent or diminished gag reflex |

Palate
(Wearing gloves)

• Lips		
• Gums	Soft, smooth	Inflammation, edema, swelling, bleeding, receding from teeth
• Tongue. Ask client to protrude tongue; grasp tip with gauze square and gently pull to each side. Palpate sides of tongue.	Muscular Nontender, smooth Pink, moist, slightly rough Midline position Voluntary movement Symmetry of shape	Induration, lesions Tender, masses, redness Fasciculations Tumors
• Teeth	Position/condition—stable, smooth	Loose, broken, irregular edges

Continued

Steps	Normal and/or Common Findings	Significant Deviations
Smell		
• Oral cavity	No odor, tobacco, smoke, food odors	Foul, acetone, alcohol odor

PEDIATRIC ADAPTATIONS

Infant

Steps	Normal and/or Common Findings	Significant Deviations
Inspection		
• Oral cavity	Pink	Thrush
	Epstein's pearls, retention cysts	
• Buccal mucosa. Note amount and	Midline uvula, freely movable	Tracheal-esophageal fistula

DENTITION

CHILD

ERUPTION OF DECIDUOUS (MILK) TEETH

UPPER	ERUPTION
CENTRAL INCISOR	5–7 MO
LATERAL INCISOR	7–10 MO
(CUSPID) CANINE	16–20 MO
FIRST MOLAR	10–16 MO
SECOND MOLAR	20–30 MO

LOWER	
SECOND MOLAR	20–30 MO
FIRST MOLAR	10–16 MO
(CUSPID) CANINE	16–20 MO
LATERAL INCISOR	8–11 MO
CENTRAL INCISOR	6–8 MO

ADULT

ERUPTION OF PERMANENT TEETH

UPPER	COMPLETED BY
CENTRAL INCISOR	9–10 YR
LATERAL INCISOR	10–11 YR
(CUSPID) CANINE	12–15 YR
FIRST PREMOLAR (BICUSPID)	12–13 YR
SECOND PREMOLAR (BICUSPID)	12–14 YR
FIRST MOLAR	6–7 YR
SECOND MOLAR	14–16 YR
THIRD MOLAR	18–25 YR

LOWER	
THIRD MOLAR	18–25 YR
SECOND MOLAR	13–16 YR
SECOND PREMOLAR (BICUSPID)	13–14 YR
FIRST PREMOLAR (BICUSPID)	12–15 YR
FIRST MOLAR	6–7 YR
(CUSPID) CANINE	10–13 YR
LATERAL INCISOR	9–10 YR
CENTRAL INCISOR	8–9 YR

FIGURE 20.
Dentition (eruption of teeth). (Source: Taber's, 17th ed., p 517 with permission.)

Steps	Normal and/or Common Findings	Significant Deviations
thickness of saliva, integrity of tissue	Small tonsils	Cleft palate, lip, or bifid uvula
		Excessive drooling in newborn
• Deciduous teeth. Note number, development, eruption dates (Fig. 20)		"Bottle mouth" — caries on lingual surfaces of all teeth
• Tongue. Note size.	Fits in mouth with teeth closed	Large, protruding
Palpate		
• Soft and hard palate	Intact	Clefts

Child

Steps	Normal and/or Common Findings	Significant Deviations
Inspection		
• Arch of palate. Note color.	Koplik's spots	
• Teeth. Note number, color.	Malocclusion at 8 years of age	
• Tonsils. Note size.	Hypertrophic in mid-childhood	Inflamed, red, edematous

Adolescent

Steps	Normal and/or Common Findings	Significant Deviations
Inspection		
• Teeth. Note presence of 2nd and 3rd molars (Fig. 20)		

GERIATRIC ADAPTATIONS

Steps	Normal and/or Common Findings	Significant Deviations
Inspection		
• Lips	Smaller, decreased fat pad	Leukoplakia, lesions, cracks in corners
• Teeth	Darkened, worn down	Multiple obvious caries, missing teeth
• Gums. Ask client to remove dentures to see gums.	May be atrophied	Irritation, lesions
• Soft and hard palate. Note color.	Pink	Lesions
• Tongue	Fissures	Extremely dry Thrush

DIAGNOSTIC TESTS

May need to refer for:
- Dental x-rays as needed
- Biopsy of suspicious lesions
- Throat cultures

POSSIBLE NURSING DIAGNOSES

- Oral mucous membarnes, altered
- Sensory-perceptual alteration: gustatory
- Nutrition, altered: less than body requirements
- Infection, high risk for
- Aspiration, high risk for

CLINICAL ALERT

- Note severe signs of dehydration if lips, mucosa, tongue are dry.
- Wear gloves to remove and clean dentures.

- Store dentures in a safe place when not in the client's mouth.
- Excess saliva may be aspirated.
- Bright red, +4 tonsils require prompt medical attention.

SAMPLE DOCUMENTATION

Oral cavity pink, moist, smooth, clean. No missing or decaying teeth. Tonsils 1+. CN IX, X, XII intact. No masses or nodules palpated.

PATIENT/FAMILY EDUCATION AND HOME HEALTH NOTES

Adult

- Brush with fluoride paste and floss between teeth at least at bedtime.

Pediatric

- Avoid prolonged exposure of mouth to milk or sweetened drinks (even before eruption of teeth). If bottle is taken to bed, it should contain only water.
- Discuss food safety with parents (e.g., aspiration, danger of straws).
- Before teeth emerge, wipe gums gently with damp, soft cloth.
- Begin brushing first tooth. May use infant toothbrush or a piece of gauze to clean teeth. See dentist between ages 1 and 2.
- Check fluoride level of drinking water for infants and children.
- Reinforce dental hygiene for the child between 7 and 10 years of age.

Geriatric

- If taste perception is decreased, encourage use of spices such as cinnamon and garlic powder instead of extra salt and sugar.

- Wear dentures most of the time to prevent atrophy of gums. See dentist if dentures do not fit and/or cause irritation or pain to gums.
- Brush and clean dentures thoroughly daily.

Lungs and Thorax

HISTORY

Adult

- Exposure to dust, chemicals and vapors, birds, asbestos, air pollutants
- Allergies. Note type, response, treatments
- Medications. Prescription and OTC
- Tobacco use. Note type, duration, amount (pack years), extent of passive smoking, years since quitting.
- History of impaired mental status
- Cough. Note causes, type, duration, severity, treatments.
- Chest pain
- Shortness of breath. Note causes, duration, treatments.
- Cyanosis or pallor
- History of emphysema, cancer, tuberculosis, heart disease, asthma, chest pain, allergies
- History of surgery, trauma
- Date of last chest x-ray and tuberculosis test
- Production of blood, other secretions with coughing

Pediatric

Infants

- Immunizations
- Respiratory distress, cyanosis, apnea
- SIDS: note whether sibling or other family member.
- Exposure to passive smoke
- History of meconium ileus

Children

- Immunizations
- Asthma history. Note associated factors related to episodes, treatment.
- Frequent colds or congestion
- Swollen lymph nodes, sore throat, facial pain
- Night coughs

Geriatric

- History of annual influenza immunization
- History of pneumonia vaccine
- Recent change in exertional capacity, fatigue
- Significant weight changes
- Change in number of pillows used at night
- Painful breathing; night sweats; swelling of hands, ankles; membranes or tingling of arms or legs; leg cramps at rest or with movement

EQUIPMENT

- Stethoscope
- Tape measure
- Pen or washable marker
- Ruler

PATIENT PREPARATION

- Sitting

PHYSICAL ASSESSMENT

Steps	Normal and/or Common Findings	Significant Deviations
Inspection		
• Shape. Note antero-posterior (AP): transverse ratio	Approximately symmetrical, AP about 0.5 diameter of transverse	Barrel chest, pigeon chest, funnel chest

Continued

Steps	Normal and/or Common Findings	Significant Deviations
• Color		Cyanosis, pallor, especially of lips, nails, gums
• Respiration. Note rate, rhythm, depth, pattern.	12–20/min Expansion symmetrical	Distress; shallow, rapid; gasping; bradypnea, tachypnea; bulging or audible sounds; retractions
• Fingers. Note shape of nails.	Uniform	Clubbing (Fig. 21)
• Lips	No effort in breathing	Pursing
• Nose	No flaring	Flaring nares
Palpation		
• Thorax. Note tenderness, motion, pulsation, crepitus.	Approximate symmetry, firm shape, nontender, elastic motion No pulsations or crepitations	Pain, tenderness Crepitus (crinkly, crackles) Friction rub (coarse vibration, usually inspiratory)
• Tactile fremitus. Place palmar surface of fingers on auscultation sites simultaneously; ask client to repeat ''99'' while palpating; compare right and left sides.	Even, symmetrical Increased over major airways, decreased over lung bases	Decreased, absent, increased asymmetrical, coarsened Crepitus
• Expansion (thumbs at 10th rib) (Fig. 22)	Symmetrical expansion of 2–3 in	Asymmetrical, expansion < 2 in
Percussion		
• Thorax. Compare left and right; note tone, intensity, pitch	(See Table 1.) Flat: large muscles, viscera, bones Dull: heart, liver Tympany: stomach Resonance: all of lung field	Hyperresonance Dullness Hyperresonance, tympany, dullness, flatness over lung tissue

Continued

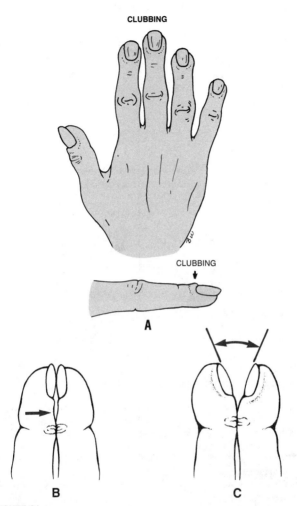

FIGURE 21.
(**A**) Clubbing of fingers. (Source: Taber's, 17th ed., p 404 with permission.)
(**B**) Normal nails with arch illustrated by arrow. (**C**) Clubbed nails with arrow illustrating loss of arch and exaggerated angle. (Source: Seidel, 2nd ed., p 113.)

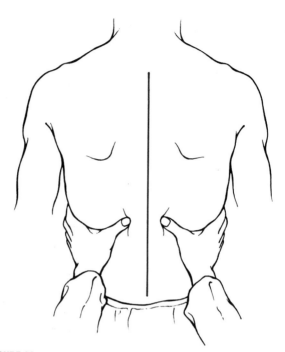

FIGURE 22.
Measurement of thoracic expansion.

Steps	Normal and/or Common Findings	Significant Deviations
• Measure diaphragmatic excursion. Percuss downward in midscapular line as client holds deep inspiration, from resonance to dullness. Mark lower border where dullness begins. Ask client to exhale	3–5 cm; may be higher on right	No change or decrease Increased excursion

Steps	Normal and/or Common Findings	Significant Deviations
completely, then percuss upward from mark to beginning of resonance. Mark and measure. Repeat on other side.		

Auscultation
• (Ask client to breathe fairly deeply through mouth.) Auscultate with diaphragm, through complete inspiration and expiration, at each site (Figs. 23, 24,	Vesicular, over lung field, inspiration > expiration; bronchovesicular over main stem bronchi, inspiration = expiration; bronchial over trachea, inspiration < expiration	Bronchovesicular or bronchial breath sounds over lung fields Diminished, absent, markedly increased breath sounds. adventitious sounds: crackles (rales),

Continued

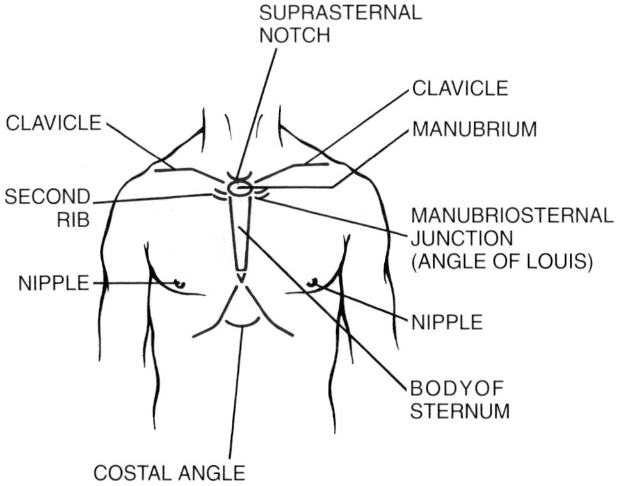

FIGURE 23.
Topographical landmarks of chest.

Steps	Normal and/or Common Findings	Significant Deviations
25) as client crosses arms over chest and leans forward. Compare bilaterally. Note pitch, intensity, duration of inspiration and expiration (Fig. 26) and any adventitious sounds (Fig. 27).		wheezes, gurgles (ronchi), friction
• Cough. Note moisture, pitch, quality, frequency.	No cough	Cough with yellow, pink, brown or gray sputum

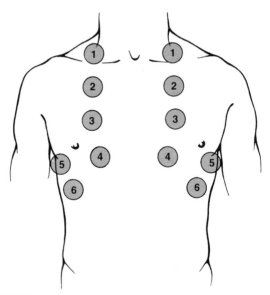

FIGURE 24.
Anterior thoracic auscultation and palpation sites.

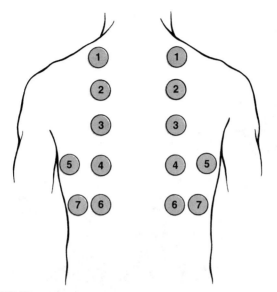

FIGURE 25.
Posterior thoracic auscultation, percussion, and palpation sites.

PEDIATRIC ADAPTATIONS

Infant

Steps	Normal and/or Common Findings	Significant Deviations
Inspection		
• Note rate.	30–60 (newborn) 22–40 (by 1 year old)	
• Shape. Note chest and head circumference.	Approximately equal in neonate	Unequal chest expansion
		Abdominal or paradoxical breathing
• Note AP and transverse diameter.	Approximately equal	

Continued

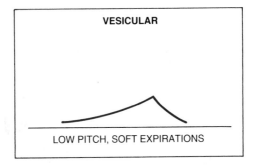

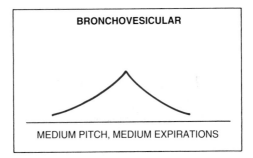

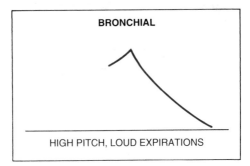

FIGURE 26.
Normal breath sounds. (Source: Adapted from Thompson, JM, et al., *Mosby's Manual of Clinical Nursing,* ed. 2, CV Mosby, St. Louis, 1989 with permission.)

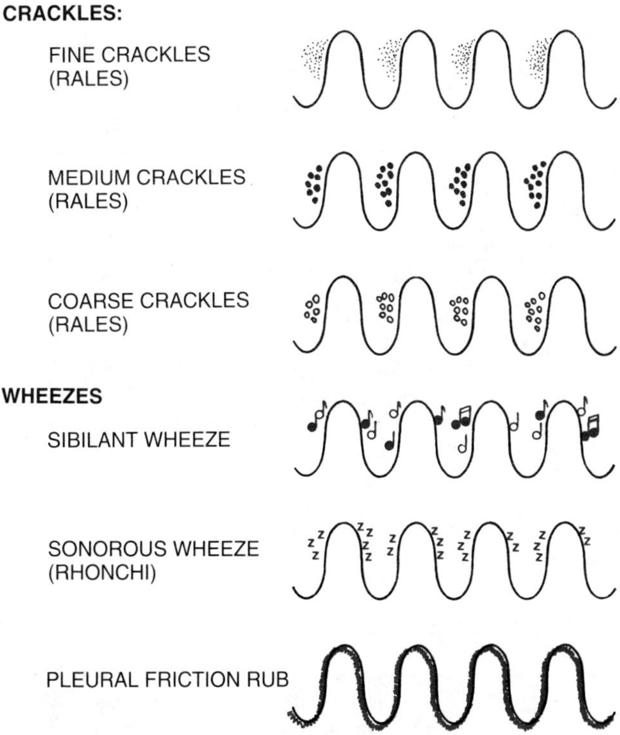

CRACKLES:

    FINE CRACKLES
    (RALES)

    MEDIUM CRACKLES
    (RALES)

    COARSE CRACKLES
    (RALES)

WHEEZES

    SIBILANT WHEEZE

    SONOROUS WHEEZE
    (RHONCHI)

    PLEURAL FRICTION RUB

FIGURE 27.
Abnormal breath sounds. (Source: Adapted from Thompson, JM, et al: *Mosby's Manual of Clinical Nursing,* ed 2, CV Mosby, St Louis, 1989 with permission.)

Steps	Normal and/or Common Findings	Significant Deviations
• Respiratory pattern	Diaphragmatic breather	Retractions, nasal flaring, periodic breathing, apnea
Auscultation		
• Lung fields	Loud, equal	Muffled, unequal, hyperresonant, diminished

Child

Steps	Normal and/or Common Findings	Significant Deviations
Inspection		
• Shape	Should approximate adult shape, uniform	Barrel chest Pectus carinatum Pectus excavatum
• Rate	Approximately 26 by age 4 20 by age 10 16 by age 16	

GERIATRIC ADAPTATIONS

Steps	Normal and/or Common Findings	Significant Deviations
Inspection		
• Thoracic spine. Note curvature, angles.	Essentially straight	Marked dorsal curvature, kyphosis, increased AP diameter of chest
• Chest expansion		Diminished

DIAGNOSTIC TESTS

May need to refer for:
- Chest x-ray
- TB tine test
- Culture and sensitivity of sputum

POSSIBLE NURSING DIAGNOSES

- Airway clearance, ineffective
- Breathing pattern, ineffective
- Suffocation, high risk for
- Tissue perfusion, altered: cardiopulmonary
- Gas exchange, impaired
- Infection, high risk for

CLINICAL ALERT

- Persistent or paroxysmal cough
- Cyanosis
- Air hunger, dyspnea
- Hemoptysis

SAMPLE DOCUMENTATION

Color pink without cyanosis or pallor. Respirations 16, regular, even depth. Chest equal symmetrically; AP diameter is half transverse. Tactile fremitus and thoracic expansion symmetrical and equal. All lung fields resonant equally. Vesicular sounds throughout; no adventitious sounds auscultated.

PATIENT/FAMILY EDUCATION AND HOME HEALTH NOTES

Adult

- Educate about smoking hazards, indoor pollution, exposure to respiratory irritants.

- Offer literature on quitting smoking, effective breathing patterns and coughing awareness, controlled breathing techniques.

Pediatric

- Educate parents regarding importance of immunizations.
- Instruct parents in risks associated with passive smoke.
- Instruct parents in safe use of vaporizer or humidifier.
- Caution parents about risks of infant/small child aspirating foreign objects, foods, and toy parts.

Geriatric

- Avoid environments where there are persons with upper respiratory infections.
- Avoid noxious fumes.
- Infection may occur without a major increase in temperature.
- Most older persons should take pneumonia and influenza vaccines.
- Raising the head and shoulders on several pillows can help persons breathe better when they feel congested.
- See physician in case of persistent cough.

Breasts and Axillae

HISTORY

Adult

- Age at menarche, menopause
- Age during pregnancies, breastfeeding
- Use of hormonal medications, oral contraceptives, hormone replacement therapy (Premarin, Estriol)
- Breast self-examination: how often, method used
- Mammogram: date, findings

- Breast surgery, trauma, or disease
- Change in breast: lumps, discharge, shape, skin, lesions, erythema swelling, tenderness, change in position of nipple, nipple discharge or inversion, relationship of breast changes to menses
- Breast cancer—self, family: age at diagnosis, treatment, response
- Lumps: size, location, how long, tenderness, relationship to menses
- Rash or eczema on nipples
- Fat and caffeine intake
- Risk factors for breast cancer:
  - Age > 40
  - Menses, early onset, late menopause
  - Nulliparity
  - Over age 30 with first pregnancy
  - Previous breast cancer
  - Ovarian, uterine, or bowel cancer
  - Medications to suppress lactation
  - Breast cancer in mother, sister, aunt, grandmother
  - High intake of dietary fat
  - Postmenopausal weight gain

Pediatric

- Age at thelarche
- Adolescent boys—unilateral or bilateral enlargement of breasts

Geriatric

- Prescription medications that may cause gynecomastia in older men
- Breast self-exams
- Recent changes in breast characteristics
- Injury to breast tissue

EQUIPMENT

- Small pillow
- Measuring tape (metric)
- Small sheet or towel

PATIENT PREPARATION

- Sitting; may need to stand and bend forward
- Maintain privacy.

PHYSICAL ASSESSMENT

Steps	Normal and/or Common Findings	Significant Deviations
Inspection		
Repeat in three positions for women, sitting position only for men: sitting arms at side; sitting, arms raised over head; sitting, hands on hips, pushing in. If breasts are very large and pendulous, have client stand, bend forward at waist; inspect for shape and contour.		
• Shape	Conical to pendulous	Marked difference in contour
• Size, symmetry	Generally equal	Marked differences
• Contour	Symmetrical	Retraction, dimpling, flattening
• Color	Light, striae	Redness

Steps	Normal and/or Common Findings	Significant Deviations
• Venous pattern	Symmetrical, faint	Superficial dilation, asymmetrically increased pattern
• Texture	Smooth, soft	Lesions, peau d'orange appearance
• Nipple, areolar tissue	Lifetime inversion, Montgomery tubercles, supernumerary nipples	Retraction, deviation, rashes, discharge, recent inversion

Palpation

Repeat in two positions for women: sitting, arms at sides; supine, small pillow under shoulder of side being palpated. Omit supine position for men. Follow either clock or wedge pattern, using pads of three fingers (Figs. 28, 29, 30). Palpate breast and axillae.		
• Consistency	Varies	Thickening, masses
• Tenderness	Tender if premenstrual	Pain
• Nodules. Note location, size, shape, consistency, delimitation, mobility, tenderness.	None	Masses, areas of induration
• Nipples (gently compress)	No discharge	Discharge

Continued

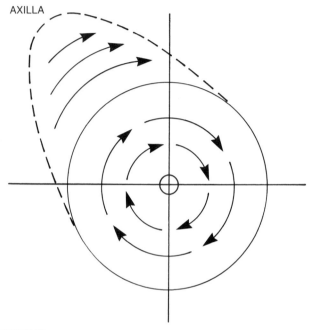

AXILLA

FIGURE 28.
A palpation method for the breast and tail of spence.

Steps	Normal and/or Common Findings	Significant Deviations
• Lymph nodes (lateral, subscapular, pectoral, central). Note presence, location, size, delimitation, shape, consistency, mobility, tenderness.	None	Palpable

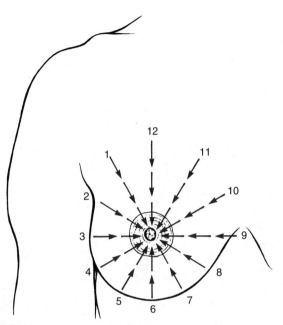

FIGURE 29.
Clock pattern of breast examination.

PEDIATRIC ADAPTATIONS
Infant

Steps	Normal and/or Common Findings	Significant Deviations
Palpation		
• Breasts. Note size, discharge.	Nonpalpable, no discharge. Engorgement < 1.5 cm, scant milky discharge in newborns; supernumerary nipples	

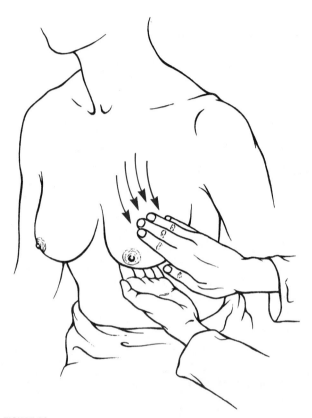

FIGURE 30.
Bimanual palpation of breast.

Child

Steps	Normal and/or Common Findings	Significant Deviations
Inspection		
• Breast. Note size, symmetry.	Breast development after age 8. May	

Steps	Normal and/or Common Findings	Significant Deviations
	be asymmetrical (see Table 3).	
Palpation		
• Breast. Note tenderness, masses.	Boys may have small, tender breast buds. Tender	Masses Gynecomastia

GERIATRIC ADAPTATIONS

Steps	Normal and/or Common Findings	Significant Deviations
Inspection		
• Breasts. Note size, shape, lesions, color, nodules.	Loose, atrophied, pendulous	Redness, irritation under breast Dimpling, flattening, masses
• Nipples. Note size, direction.	Flat, small	

TABLE 3
STAGES OF SECONDARY SEXUAL CHARACTERISTICS

Stage	Female Breast Development
I	Preadolescent—elevation of papilla only
II	Small breast bud—elevation of breast and nipple with enlarging areola
III	Areola and breast tissue enlarged
IV	Areola and papillae form secondary—contour develops simultaneous mound on breast
V	Maturity

Source: Data from Tanner, J. M.: *Growth at Adolescence,* ed 2. Blackwell Scientific Publications, Oxford, England, 1962.

DIAGNOSTIC TESTS

May need to refer for:
- Mammogram
- Biopsy

POSSIBLE NURSING DIAGNOSES

- Tissue integrity, impaired
- Body image disturbance
- Self-esteem disturbance
- Anxiety

CLINICAL ALERT

- Refer any suspicious lump or any recent change

SAMPLE DOCUMENTATION

No history of breast disease; performs BSE monthly. Breasts symmetrical, small, without lesions; texture smooth. No discharge or tenderness of nipple or areola. No masses or tenderness palpable in any region of breast, tail. No axillary or epitrochlear nodes palpable.

PATIENT EDUCATION/HOME HEALTH NOTES

Adult

- Instruct (males and females) in BSE (Fig. 31).
- Explain effects of large intake of caffeine on breasts.
- Explain importance of mammogram and suggested schedule: once between ages 35 to 40; every year or every other year ages 40 to 50; every year after age 50 (more frequently if at risk).

Pediatric

Infants

- Explain influence of maternal hormones to parents if infant has palpable breast tissue.

BREAST SELF-EXAMINATION

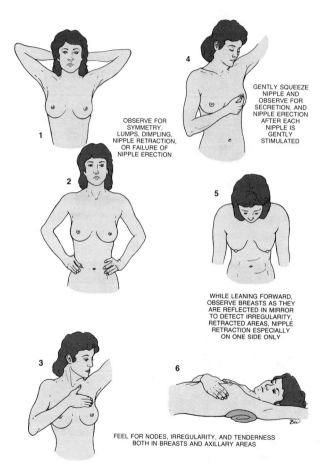

OBSERVE FOR SYMMETRY, LUMPS, DIMPLING, NIPPLE RETRACTION, OR FAILURE OF NIPPLE ERECTION

GENTLY SQUEEZE NIPPLE AND OBSERVE FOR SECRETION, AND NIPPLE ERECTION AFTER EACH NIPPLE IS GENTLY STIMULATED

WHILE LEANING FORWARD, OBSERVE BREASTS AS THEY ARE REFLECTED IN MIRROR TO DETECT IRREGULARITY, RETRACTED AREAS, NIPPLE RETRACTION ESPECIALLY ON ONE SIDE ONLY

FEEL FOR NODES, IRREGULARITY, AND TENDERNESS BOTH IN BREASTS AND AXILLARY AREAS

FIGURE 31.
Breast self-examination. (Source: Taber's, 17th ed., p 266 with permission.)

Children

- Explain patterns of breast development.
- Reassure adolescent boys with breast enlargement that condition is temporary.
- Teach BSE.

Geriatric

- Monthly BSE at set date every month after menopause (for example, the first day of the month)

Cardiovascular

HISTORY

Adult

- Tobacco use: age started, type, amount (pack years), duration, years since quitting
- Exercise habits: amount, type, duration, response
- Nutrition: usual diet; fat, salt, cholesterol, calorie intake
- Weight, recent change, percent obese
- Alcohol use: amount, frequency
- Stress management skills, ability, and methods used to relax; response to pressure, anger
- Self or family history of heart disease, diabetes, rheumatic fever, hyperlipidemia, hypertension, early deaths
- Presence or history of chest pain: onset, duration, severity, characteristics, associated symptoms, treatment, response
- Shortness of breath
- Recent increase in fatigue, inability to complete usual activities
- Dyspnea, orthopnea
- Cough
- Leg cramps: onset (daily activities, awake at night), duration, characteristics
- Extremities: coldness, tingling, numbness, cyanosis, lesions, varicosities, slowed healing, edema
- Medication use: prescription and OTC

Pediatric

Infants

- Unusual fatigue or effort, especially when sucking
- Circumoral cyanosis
- Coordination problems
- Generalized cyanosis (especially when crying)

Children

- Unusual fatigue. Note amount, degree, activity level, need for rest.
- Assumption of squatting or knee-chest position when playing
- Difficulty feeding
- Complaints of leg pain, joint pain, headache.
- Nosebleeds
- Frequent streptococcal infections or sore throat with fever

Geriatric

- Chest pain, chest pressure, chest tightness
- Unusual fatigue, increased need for rest
- Orthopnea; note number of pillows
- Shortness of breath, dyspnea, coughing, wheezing
- Dizziness, syncope, palpitations, confusion
- Use of cardiac or hypertensive medications
- Pounding heart with stress
- Dietary history: note intake of potassium, cholesterol, caffeine
- Nocturia
- Foot and leg edema (tightness of shoes at end of day)
- Change in exercise level
- Use of restrictive clothing
- Shortness of breath at night
- Peripheral vascular complaints such as coldness, decreased pain sensation, exaggerated response to cold

EQUIPMENT

- Stethoscope with diaphragm and bell
- Centimeter ruler

- Light
- Scale

(The assessment of blood pressure is a part of the cardiac system but is found in the vital signs section.)

PATIENT PREPARATION

- Remove clothing, drape well for warmth and privacy.
- Positions: primarily sitting; also supine, left lateral recumbent, standing

PHYSICAL ASSESSMENT—HEART

Steps	Normal and/or Common Findings	Significant Deviations
Inspection		
• Precordium movement with tangential lighting	Slight apical impulse at MCL, 5th ICS	Marked pulsation; often not visible; impulse visible in more than one ICS or lateral to MCL; pulsations in other locations; heaves, lifts
• Jugular vein		
• General muscle mass		
Palpation		
• Lightly palpate precordium. Note location, strength of apical impulse.	Mild sensation palpable at 5th LICS, MCL	Thrills, pulsations Palpable in radius > 1–2 cm or significantly to left or right of MCL or upward
• Palpate carotid and apical impulse simultaneously.	Synchronous pulses	

Steps	Normal and/or Common Findings	Significant Deviations
Auscultation		
• Auscultate in each of five areas (Fig. 32). Sitting, with diaphragm; supine, with both diaphragm and bell	Synchronous pulses	
• Note rate, rhythm, location, and nature of S_1, S_2.	Normal sinus rhythm. S_1 loudest at apex. S_2 at base. Splitting of S_1 usually heard at left lower sternal border (tricuspid area); split-	S_3, S_4 audible at apex on inspiration Extra heart sounds such as clicks, snaps, friction rubs

Continued

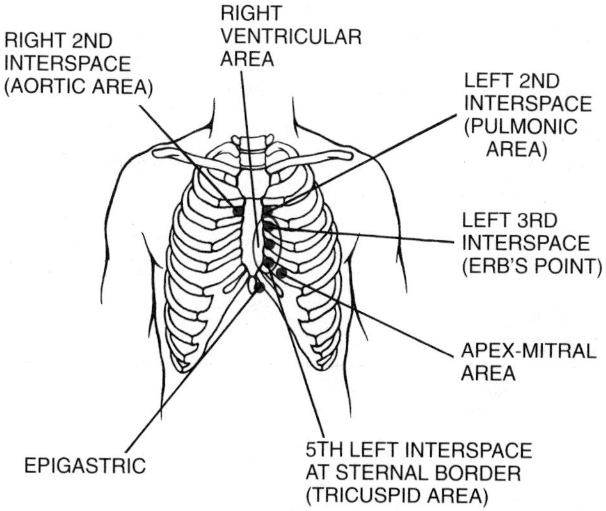

RIGHT 2ND INTERSPACE (AORTIC AREA)

RIGHT VENTRICULAR AREA

LEFT 2ND INTERSPACE (PULMONIC AREA)

LEFT 3RD INTERSPACE (ERB'S POINT)

APEX-MITRAL AREA

5TH LEFT INTERSPACE AT STERNAL BORDER (TRICUSPID AREA)

EPIGASTRIC

FIGURE 32.
Cardiac auscultation and palpation sites.

Steps	Normal and/or Common Findings	Significant Deviations
	ting of S_2 usually heard during inspiration at 2nd or 3rd LICS.	
• Auscultate along left sternal border at 2nd and 3rd ICS (pulmonic area) with bell as client leans forward. With client in left lateral recumbent position, auscultate at 5th LICS (mitral area) with bell.	No murmurs	Murmurs audible. Note if increased on inspiration or expiration, with Valsalva maneuver, with elevation of legs, or if associated with diastole or systole. (See Table 4.)

PHYSICAL ASSESSMENT—PERIPHERAL CIRCULATION

Steps	Normal and/or Common Findings	Significant Deviations
Inspection		
• Skin of extremities. Note color, continuity, edema, vascularity.	Pink, no edema, no lesions	Cyanosis, lesions, ulcers, varicosities, edema, rubor

TABLE 4
CLASSIFICATION OF MURMURS

Classification	Murmur
Grade I	Faint
Grade II	Heard fairly well in all positions
Grade III	Loud, no thrills
Grade IV	Loud, with a thrill
Grade V	Very loud, easily palpable thrill
Grade VI	May be heard without a stethoscope, thrill present

Steps	Normal and/or Common Findings	Significant Deviations
Palpation		
• Palpate carotid pulses (one at a time).	Symmetrical, rate 60–100 bpm, regular rhythm	Unequal, marked bradycardia, tachycardia, arrhythmias such as bigeminal pulse, alternating pulse, trigeminal pulse, bounding or absent pulse
• Palpate peripheral pulses bilaterially: ◦ Brachial ◦ Radial ◦ Femoral ◦ Popliteal ◦ Dorsalis pedis ◦ Posterior tibial. Note rate, rhythm, strength, symmetry; compare side to side.		
• Palpate extremities. Note temperature, tenderness, turgor, texture, hair growth, nails, varicosities, lesions, capillary refill time.	Warm; nontender; firm without edema, equal, fine hair growth. No lesions or varicosities.	Cool, tender, pitting edema (0 to +4), absence of hair, varicose veins
• Measure jugular venous pressure. Place client in supine position with 45° elevation of head and shoulders. Observe jugular pulsation. With centimeter ruler, measure between highest point of	≤ 2 cm; usually absent in persons < 50 years	> 2 cm

Continued

Steps	Normal and/or Common Findings	Significant Deviations
jugular pulsation and angle of Louis (Fig. 33). Mark the jugular pressure point with a straightedge for ease of measuring. Repeat on other side.		
Auscultation • Auscultate with bell: temporal, carotid.	No audible sounds	Bruits

PEDIATRIC ADAPTATIONS

Infant

Steps	Normal and/or Common Findings	Significant Deviations
Inspection • Apical impulse. Note location.	4th LICS medial to MCL ($<$ 5 years)	
Palpation • Apical impulse		Thrills
• Femoral and brachial pulses. Note symmetry.	Equal bilaterally	
• Note capillary refill.	1–2 seconds	$>$ 2 seconds
Auscultation • Heart sounds. Note rate, rhythm, location, nature of S_1, S_2, S_3.	Louder, higher pitched, shorter duration, 110–160 bpm, sinus arrhythmia	Machinelike continuous murmur, bradycardia, tachycardia

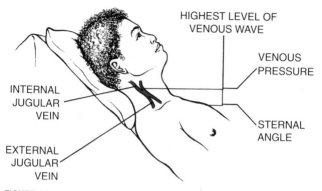

FIGURE 33.
Inspection of jugular vein.

Child

Steps	Normal and/or Common Findings		Significant Deviations
Inspection			
• Apical impulse medial to left MCL at 4th ICS in child < 5 years old	1 year	80–140	
	3 years	80–120	
	5 years	75–110	
	10 years	70–100	
	Sinus arrhythmia		
Auscultation			
• Heart sounds	Splitting of S_2 at apex; innocent murmurs grade 3 or less, present in systole, varying with respirations, found along left sternal border with child supine		No splitting of S_2 during inspiration

GERIATRIC ADAPTATIONS

Steps	Normal and/or Common Findings	Significant Deviations
Inspection		
• Feet, toes	Gradual pink or purple discoloration common Nails thicken. Hair thins.	Rubor, lesions, marked edema, persistent cyanosis
Auscultation		
• Blood pressure	Pulse pressure may reach 100	Varies, serial readings > 170/95
• Heart sounds	Arrhythmias are common. Murmurs may be benign, due to stiffened valves. S_4 may be due to decreased left ventricle compliance.	S_3S_4

DIAGNOSTIC TESTS

May need to refer for:
• Cardiac catheterization
• Exercise stress test
• Chest x-ray
• Enzyme studies
• ECG
• CBC
• Triglycerides
• Cholesterol

POSSIBLE NURSING DIAGNOSES

• Nutrition, altered: high risk for more than body requirements
• Skin integrity, impaired, high risk for

- Cardiac output, decreased
- Tissue perfusion, altered
- Activity intolerance
- Fatigue
- Sensory-perceptual alterations
- Self-care deficit
- Role preformance, altered
- Knowledge deficit

CLINICAL ALERT

- Refer any unusual heart sounds.
- Report decreased circulation, venous insufficiency.
- Refer chest pain, dyspnea, marked hypertension immediately.

SAMPLE DOCUMENTATION

BP 126/72, apical pulse 80, RRR, PMI at 5th interspace. Extremities symmetrically warm, pink, without edema or clubbing; peripheral pulses equally palpable (carotid, radial, femoral, popliteal, posterior tibial, dorsalis pedis).

PATIENT/FAMILY EDUCATION AND HOME HEALTH NOTES

Adult

- Discuss risk factors of heart disease.
- Explain principles of aerobic exercise and low-fat, low-cholesterol diet in prevention of heart disease.
- Offer guidelines on stress management, including minimal use of caffeine, tobacco, and alcohol.
- Explain importance of unrestricted circulation: include regular exercise; avoid sitting for prolonged periods; elevate legs if necessary to sit for prolonged period; avoid tight clothing, especially socks and hosiery; avoid crossed legs while sitting.

Pediatric

- Explain to parents the importance of lifetime habits for good nutrition and exercise.
- Stress the need for fats in the infant's and toddler's diet, then teach parents to reduce fats in the child's diet.
- Discuss possible need for additional iron during infancy and adolescence.

Geriatric

- Check with physician before starting an exercise program. Stop exercising when you feel tired.
- Review medications and provide appropriate education, including need to take medications as prescribed.
- Teach about importance of proper foot care.
- Report any new shortness of breath and/or edema to physician.
- Monitor blood pressure.
- Teach how to check blood pressure and pulse rate.

Abdomen

HISTORY

Adult

- Appetite
- Diet recall for the past 24 hours
- Dysphagia
- Weight gain or loss
- Use of alcohol, tobacco, caffeine (duration, amount, frequency)
- Bowel/bladder routines, problems
- Indigestion, nausea, vomiting, pain, jaundice, flatulence (causes, frequency, treatments)
- Pain (type, predisposing factors, time)
- Medications for bowel, indigestion

- History of hepatitis, ulcer, arthritis
- History of gastrointestinal diagnostic tests, surgery

Pediatric

- Jaundice
- Pain or paroxysmal fussiness and intense crying
- Frequent spitting-up
- Projectile vomiting
- Constipation, encopresis, crying while urinating, frequency of urinary tract infections (UTI)
- Introduction to new foods
- Type and methods of feeding
- Parental concerns
- Milk intake
- Pica intake

Geriatric

- Abdominal pain, specifying whether the pain is associated with eating
- Excessive belching; bloating; flatulence
- Changes in appetite (especially a decrease in appetite)
- Nausea; vomiting; diarrhea
- Hemorrhoids, changes in bowel habits
- Rectal bleeding, pain, itching; hernia

EQUIPMENT

- Ink pen
- Stethoscope
- Tape measure
- Gloves

PATIENT PREPARATION

- Have patient empty bladder
- Lying on back with knees bent

- Have parent hold child < 3 years on lap if unable to lie on back

PHYSICAL ASSESSMENT

Steps	Normal and/or Common Findings	Significant Deviations
Inspection		
• Shape. Note symmetry, contour.	Flat, rounded	Protuberant, scaphoid (Fig. 34), asymmetry, masses
• Color	Same as or lighter than other areas	Redness, cyanosis, jaundice, lesions (see Integumentary System)
• Surface. Note motion (respiratory, digestive).		Circulatory pulsations Dilated veins
Auscultation		
Lightly place warmed stethoscope diaphragm.		
• Abdomen. Note bowel sounds: pitch, volume, frequency in four quadrants (Fig. 35).	Bowel sounds, 5–35/ minute No vascular sounds	No bowel sounds, absence of borborygmus Bruits, hums, rubs
• Aortic, renal, femoral, arteries		

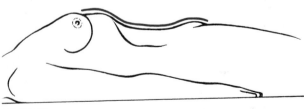

FIGURE 34.
Scaphoid abdomen.

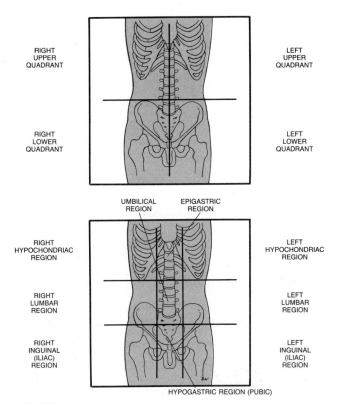

FIGURE 35.
Abdominal quadrants and regions. (Source: Taber's, 17th ed., p 4 with permission.)

Steps	Normal and/or Common Findings	Significant Deviations
Percussion • Four quadrants. Note percussion sounds (see Table 1).	Tympany, dullness	

Continued

Steps	Normal and/or Common Findings	Significant Deviations
• Liver. Note size. On right mid-clavicular line (MCL), percuss upward from waist to dullness (lower border). Mark with pen at dullness. Move up to lung resonance and percuss downward in MCL to dullness (upper border of liver). Mark at dullness and measure (Fig. 36).	6–12 cm	Enlarged > 12 cm or < 6 cm
• Spleen. Note size. Percuss on left side, distal to MCL (have patient turn slightly to right side).	Should be between ribs 6 and 10	Enlarged

Palpation

Use the palmar surface of extended fingers.

• Abdominal wall (palpate lightly)	No tenderness, pain, masses	Tenderness, rigidity, nodules
• Abdominal wall (palpate deeply) (Fig. 37). Check four quadrants (see Fig. 35).		Tenderness, masses, bulges
• Note organs (liver, spleen, kidneys).		
• Aorta	Palpable in midline	Prominent lateral pulsation

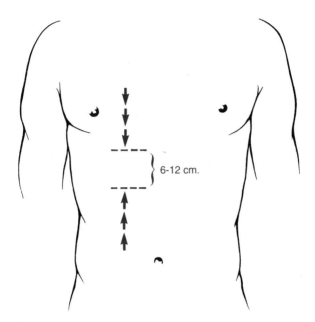

FIGURE 36.
Percussion of liver.

PEDIATRIC ADAPTATIONS

Neonate

Steps	Normal and/or Common Findings	Significant Deviations
Inspection		
• Shape of abdomen	Flat immediately following birth, then prominent and protuberant	Scaphoid abdomen in neonate may indicate diaphragmatic hernia.

Continued

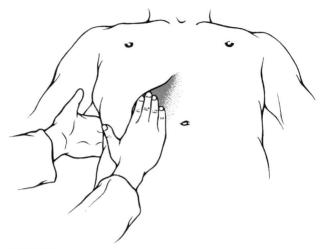

FIGURE 37.
Liver palpation.

Steps	Normal and/or Common Findings	Significant Deviations
• Umbilical cord	Presence of two umbilical arteries, thick white or cream colored walls, and one vein	One umbilical artery

Infant

Steps	Normal and/or Common Findings	Significant Deviations
Inspection		
• Shape of abdomen	Protuberant because of the underdevel-	Herniations: diastasis recti; weakness of

Steps	Normal and/or Common Findings	Significant Deviations
	oped musculature	the musculature, umbilical or ventral
• Motion		Visible reverse peristalsis
• Umbilical stump. Note color, odor.	Stump falls off 10–15 days after birth.	Signs of infection; foul odor
Auscultation		
• Bowel sounds	Hear every 10–30 seconds.	Absent, hyperactive
Palpation		
Have infant supine; place folded blanket under infant's knees and hips to elevate feet and relax abdominal muscles. Because infants have limited verbal ability, observe infant for facial cues indicating discomfort.		Olive-shaped mass in RUQ
• Liver	1–2 cm below right costal margin (RCM)	Enlarged
• Spleen tip		
• Bladder		
• Descending colon		Tenderness, mass, difficult to assess
Percussion		
• Bladder	May reach level of umbilicus at times	
• Stomach	Children have more tympany than adults because of presence of more air in intestines.	

Child

Steps	Normal and/or Common Findings	Significant Deviations
Inspection		
• Shape of abdomen	Abdomen should be protuberant when child is standing, flat when lying supine	
• Abdomen. Note pulsations.		Marked aortic pulsation
Palpation Place child's hand under yours to prevent tickling.		
• Liver edge	Should be less than 3 cm below costal margin	Child keeps knees drawn up, abdominal pain, splinting abdomen Enlarged liver
• Bladder	May be palpated just above the symphysis pubis in the preschooler	
• Spleen tip	1–2 cm: below LCM	Enlarged spleen
• Lower poles of both kidneys		

GERIATRIC ADAPTATIONS

Steps	Normal and/or Common Findings	Significant Deviations
Inspection		
• Contour	Sagging, rounded because of loss of muscle tone and an increase in fat deposits	

Steps	Normal and/or Common Findings	Significant Deviations
Palpation		
• Liver. Note size.	May be decreased but may extend 2–3 cm below right costal margin because of enlarged lung fields	
• Aorta	May be dilated	
Auscultation		
• Bowel sounds	Diminished peristalsis Hyperactive with large doses of laxatives	Absent

DIAGNOSTIC TESTS

May need to refer for:
- CBC
- Alkaline phosphatase
- Bilirubin
- Electrolytes
- Barium enema
- Chest x-ray
- Urinalysis
- Guaiac test

POSSIBLE NURSING DIAGNOSES

- Constipation, perceived or colonic
- Diarrhea
- Urinary elimination, altered patterns of
- Fluid volume deficit, active loss
- Nutrition, altered, less than or more than body requirements
- Sleep pattern disturbance

CLINICAL ALERT

- Absence of bowel sounds
- Palpable masses
- Enlarged spleen, liver
- Acute abdominal pain

SAMPLE DOCUMENTATION

Abdomen smooth, rounded, without visible motions of digestion, circulation. Bowel sounds auscultated in all quadrants. Liver size approximately 10 cm at MCL, not palpable. No other organs or masses palpated, no tenderness.

PATIENT/FAMILY EDUCATION AND HOME HEALTH NOTES

Adult

- Explain components of balanced diet—calories/height/activity; one formula: ideal weight × 13–15–20 activity factor; ≤ 30% fats (10% each: saturated, monounsaturated, polyunsaturated); cholesterol < 300 mg daily; 12% protein; 48% carbohydrates; ≤ 10% refined sugar; salt ≤ 5 g daily

Pediatric

- Explain goals of basic nutrition to parents.
- Encourage offering wide variety of nutritious foods to child and *not* offering empty calories such as soft drinks, candy, pastries.
- Explain toddler-preschool eating patterns, i.e., food jags, strong preference for only a few foods. Teach parents to assess diet over several days rather than one meal.
- Discuss the need for fat in the infant's and toddler's diet.

Geriatric

- Teach techniques to prevent constipation: daily exercise, fluids to 2,000 ml/day, whole grains and fiber in diet such as vegetables (broccoli and cauliflower) and prunes.

Musculoskeletal

HISTORY

Adult

- Client's age
- LMP or years since menopause
- Weight
- Height, loss of height
- Tobacco use
- Ability to care for self
- Exercise patterns, equipment
- Knowledge and use of good body mechanics
- Assess dietary calcium, vitamin D, protein intake
- History of joint pain, swelling, heat, arthritis, bone injury
- Muscular pain, tremors, stiffness
- Weakness
- Joint, bone, muscle trauma
- Use of hormone replacement therapy
- Medications (anti-inflammatory agents, aspirin)
- Self or family history of osteoporosis, arthritis, muscle disease, tuberculosis

Pediatric

Infant

- Birth injuries, macrosomia
- Alignment of hips, knees, ankles
- Trauma

Children

- Participation in sports, outdoor activities
- Frequent contact or high impact fractures, limping, complaints of aches or pain in joints, other trauma

Geriatric

- Stiffness, backache
- History of injuries (fractures, dislocations, whiplash)

- Weakness or pain with muscle use (location/weakness and activity altered)
- Problems with manual dexterity
- Deformity or coordination difficulties
- Problems with shoes
- Restless legs; transient paresthesia
- Alterations in gait (weakness, balance problems, difficulty with steps, fear of falling)
- Walking aids
- Joint swelling, pain, redness, heat, deformity, stiffness (pronounced at certain times of day, or associated with or following activity/inactivity)
- Limited movement (specify)
- Crepitation
- Interference with ADL

EQUIPMENT

- Tape measure
- Goniometer

PATIENT PREPARATION

- Sitting
- Supine
- Standing (balance)
- Walking (observation of gait)

PHYSICAL ASSESSMENT

Steps	Normal and/or Common Findings	Significant Deviations
Inspection		
• Posture. Note symmetry, erectness.	Erect, flexible, mobile, slumped, rounded shoulders	Spinal curvatures (see below) Legs of uneven length

Steps	Normal and/or Common Findings	Significant Deviations
• Major muscle groups. Note symmetry.	Atrophy, mild hypertrophy Bilateral symmetry	Marked or unexplained hypertrophy, asymmetry Marked or unexplained atrophy
• Joints. Note color: neck, shoulder, elbow, wrist, hip, knee, ankle, foot (Figs. 38, 39, 40, 41).	Full ROM	Edema, redness, heat, limitation in motion, deformities
• Spine. Have client bend at waist.	Full ROM	Curvature Kyphosis (Fig. 42) Scoliosis Lordosis
Palpation		
• Joints. Note mobility, ROM, symmetry, temperature.	Full active and passive ROM	Tenderness, warmth, edema, stiffness, instability
• Muscles. Note tone, strength by having client resist pressure; compare bilaterally.	Firm, tense on movement Strength 3 to 4+	Soft, flabby Weakness 1+

PEDIATRIC ADAPTATIONS

Infant

Steps	Normal and/or Common Findings	Significant Deviations
Inspection		
• Muscle tone	Taut	Decreased muscle tone

Continued

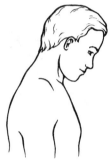
FLEXION

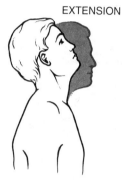
EXTENSION

HYPEREXTENSION

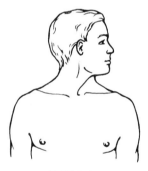
ROTATION

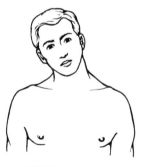
LATERAL FLEXION

FIGURE 38.
Range of motion of neck.

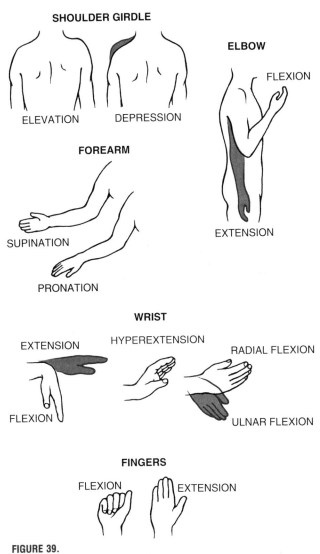

FIGURE 39.
Range of motion of upper extremity.

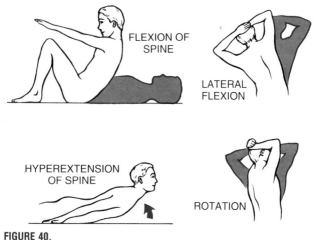

FIGURE 40.
Range of motion of trunk.

Steps	Normal and/or Common Findings	Significant Deviations
• Feet, legs. Note tibial torsion and/or metatarsus adductus; if present, use gentle pressure in attempt to straighten foot.	Tibial torsion should resolve after 6 months	Polydactyly or syndactyly Inability to straighten foot
Palpation		
• Clavicles	Intact	Fractures or absent
• Hips	Equal gluteal folds, equal movement	Ortolani's sign (dislocation) (Fig. 43) Barlow's sign Unequal gluteal folds, limited ROM

Continued

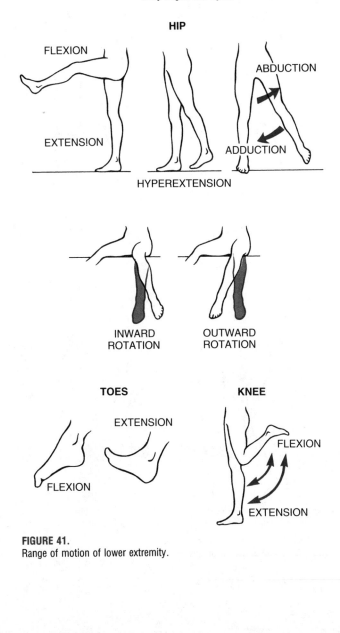

FIGURE 41.
Range of motion of lower extremity.

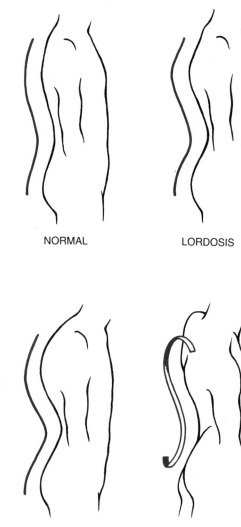

NORMAL

LORDOSIS

KYPHOSIS

SCOLIOSIS

FIGURE 42.
Normal and abnormal spinal curves.

A

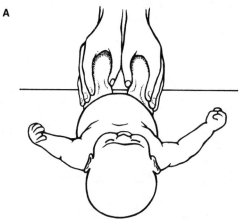

STEP 1

B

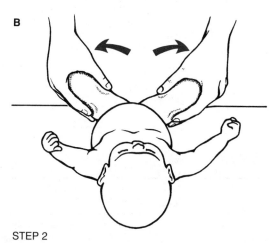

STEP 2

FIGURE 43.
Hip dislocation in infant.

Steps	Normal and/or Common Findings	Significant Deviations
• Spine	Intact, smooth	Defects in vertebral column, dimples, or hair tufts
• ROM	Full in all joints but may resist	
• Muscles. Note bilateral strength.	May elicit Moro response	Hypertonicity, flaccidity

Child

Steps	Normal and/or Common Findings	Significant Deviations
Inspection		
• Legs	Genu varum and metatarsus adductus (normal to age 2)	Asymmetry Toeing-in
• Knees	Genu valgum (from ages 2–10)	More than 2½ in between malleolus when knees are touching
• Spine	Increased lumbar curvature in toddlers	Scoliosis

GERIATRIC ADAPTATIONS

Steps	Normal and/or Common Findings	Significant Deviations
Inspection (Client sitting)		
• Spine	Kyphosis	Severe kyphosis
• Joints of fingers, hands, wrists, shoulders, elbows, knees, ankles, toes	Limitation in normal ROM, instability	Swelling, nodules, heat, redness, crepitus, deformities (Fig. 44)

Continued

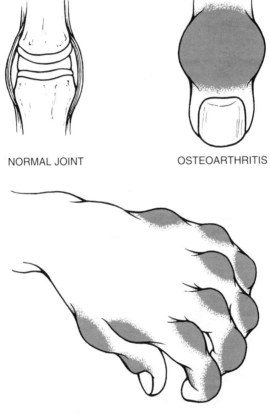

NORMAL JOINT   OSTEOARTHRITIS

RHEUMATOID ARTHRITIS

FIGURE 44.

Steps	Normal and/or Common Findings	Significant Deviations
• Muscles	Decreased muscle mass	
• Feet	Corns, calluses, hammertoes, bunions	
(Client standing)		
• Spine. Note ROM, symmetry, posture.	Abnormal curvature, especially kyphosis. Slowed movement, diminished sense of balance. Diminished muscle mass and strength bilaterally	Severe kyphosis
Test		
(Client sitting)		
• ROM. Check neck, fingers, hands, wrists, shoulders, elbows.	Diminished joint flexibility bilaterally	
• ROM. Check ankles, feet, knees, hips.	Diminished joint flexibility bilaterally	

DIAGNOSTIC TESTS

May need to refer for:
- Bone x-ray to detect osteoporosis
- Blood tests for rheumatoid factor, calcium, and uric acid

POSSIBLE NURSING DIAGNOSES

- Injury, high risk for
- Physical mobility, impaired
- Sleep pattern disturbance
- Protection, altered
- Activity intolerance, high risk for

- Fatigue
- Self-care deficit: toileting
- Chronic pain
- Disuse syndrome, high risk for

CLINICAL ALERT

- Protect older clients from falling
- Prevent contractures by exercise and ROM activities

SAMPLE DOCUMENTATION

Posture relaxed, erect; no lordosis, kyphosis, scoliosis visible. Joints mobile, nontender; full ROM demonstrated in every joint. Muscle strength and size equal bilaterally.

PATIENT/FAMILY EDUCATION AND HOME HEALTH NOTES

Adult

- Maintain muscle strength and joint flexibility through exercise.
- Teach appropriate exercise techniques.
- Teach risk factors associated with osteoporosis (sedentary life-style, poor dietary calcium, female, small-boned, low weight, white, fair-skinned, smoking, heavy alcohol use). Encourage prevention beginning in youth, extending through lifetime.
- Teach safety risks associated with falls in home, such as loose rugs, poor lighting, uneven surfaces, wet surfaces (tub, bathroom floor).

Pediatric

- Encourage physical fitness early with regular exercise.
- See Adult (above). Teach parents and adolescent about prevention of osteoporosis as well as maintenance of mobility.
- Teach safety at home.

Geriatric

- Teach proper diet and exercise to reduce progression of osteoporosis.
- Help plan specific exercise program: 20 minutes three times a week after checking with physician.
- Teach:
  - Techniques to control chronic pain
  - Correct use of assistive devices
  - Prevention of immobility
  - Safety measures (e.g., adequate lighting, removal of throw rugs)

Neurologic

HISTORY

Adult

- Headaches
- Dizziness
- Visual disturbances
- Numbness, weakness, spasms
- Twitching, tremors
- Forgetfulness
- History of head injury, nerve injury, seizures, syncope
- Changes in senses of taste, smell, hearing
- Difficulty swallowing
- Speech difficulties
- Seizures
- Change in cognition, behavior, communication, memory
- Use of all medications (antidepressants, anticonvulsants, antivertigo agents)
- Use of alcohol or mood-altering medications
- Exposure to chemicals, pesticides

Pediatric

Infant

- Apgar score of infant
- Birth trauma; other trauma
- Maternal alcohol or substance abuse
- Maternal or neonatal exposure to TORCH viruses
- Dietary intake for 24 hours
- Patterns of behavior and daily schedule

Child

- Past head injuries, illnesses, fevers
- Attainment of developmental milestones: head control, sits, crawls, walks, speaks, fine motor control
- Change in behavior, personality, cognition, communication
- Daily schedule, preschool, games
- Fever, projectile vomiting
- Amount and type of television viewed
- Interactions
- Use of drugs
- Neck stiffness, high-pitched cry

Geriatric

- Sensory disturbances (paresthesia, hyperesthesia, diplopia)
- Dizziness, faintness, spells, attacks, weakness; headaches
- Changes in gait, coordination and balance; vertigo
- History of injuries or falls, particularly recent ones
- Mental status changes such as in mood, thinking process, or cognitive process
- Speech alterations
- How any symptoms affect ADL

EQUIPMENT

- Tuning fork
- Reflex hammer

- Cotton balls
- Familiar object (coin, paper clip, button)
- Sharp object

PATIENT PREPARATION

- Sitting
- Standing

PHYSICAL ASSESSMENT

Steps	Normal and/or Common Findings	Significant Deviations
	MOTOR/SENSORY	
Inspection		
• Extremities. Note coordination, gait, tremor.	Smooth motions, no tremor	Tremor; abnormal gaits such as shuffling
• Large muscles. Note symmetrical size, involuntary movements.	No involuntary movement	
	Symmetrical (muscles of dominant side may be slightly larger).	
Test		
• Romberg. Have client stand with both eyes open, then closed, with arms at sides, feet together (20–30 seconds). Stand near client in case balance is lost.	Minimal or no swaying	Drift, imbalance
Palpation		
• Extremities. Note touch perception (with cotton ball),	Equal perception of vibration	Absent or asymmetrical vibratory perception

Steps	Normal and/or Common Findings	Significant Deviations
vibratory perception (with tuning fork over bone) Distinguish between sharp and dull.		
• Large muscles. Note symmetrical strength against resistance.	Symmetrical	Unequal weakness

REFLEXES

Test		
• Biceps, triceps, brachioradialis, patellar knee jerk, Achilles, plantar (Figs. 45, 46, 47) using percussion hammer (Fig. 48)	+2	Diminished or increased responses

COGNITION/MENTAL STATUS

(See Appendix D)

Test		
• Orientation to person, place, time	Oriented × 3	Unable to orient self, setting, date
• Memory. Note immediate, recent, and remote recall.	Intact	Memory loss of significant immediate or recent events
• Affect and mood	Appropriate to setting and circumstance	Inappropriate emotional response
• Judgment and ability to abstract	Responds appropriately	Judgment impaired
• Thought content and process		Inappropriate

Continued

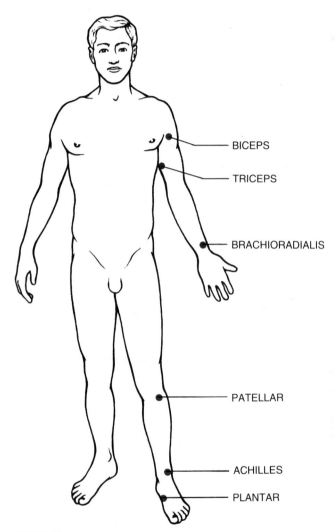

FIGURE 45.
Reflexes.

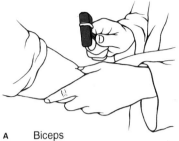

A Biceps

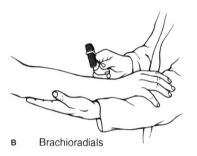

B Brachioradials

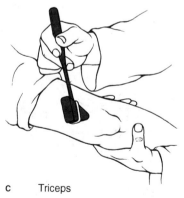

C Triceps

FIGURE 46.
Eliciting deep tendon reflexes.

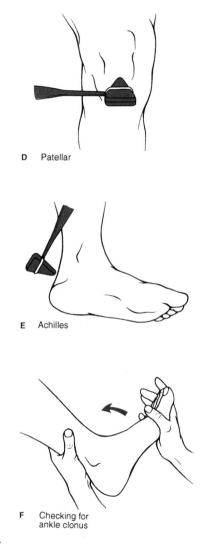

D   Patellar

E   Achilles

F   Checking for
      ankle clonus

FIGURE 46.
Continued.

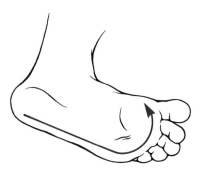

FIGURE 47.
Eliciting the plantar reflex.

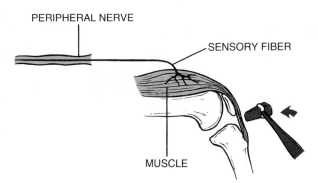

PERIPHERAL NERVE

SENSORY FIBER

MUSCLE

FIGURE 48.
Use of percussion hammer to elicit reflex response.

Steps	Normal and/or Common Findings	Significant Deviations
	CRANIAL NERVES	
(See Table 5)		
Test (If not tested with above systems)		
• CN I: ability to identify odors	Appropriate and symmetrical response for each Able to smell	Absent or asymmetrical response
• CN II: visual acuity	Able to see	
• CN III: pupils, EOMS	Pupils constrict, eyes move through fields symmetrically.	Asymmetrical pupillary response. Nystagmus
• CN IV: lid movements		
• CN V: facial sensation, muscle strength, corneal reflexes	Equal sensation and strength Blink symmetrical	Decreased or absent sensation; absent blink
• CN VI: lateral eye movements	Even eye movements	
• CN VII: facial muscle strength, taste	Symmetrical strength	Drooping lid Paralysis Decreased strength
• CN VIII: hearing acuity, sound conduction	Equal acuity	Hearing loss
• CN IX: taste, gag reflex	Voice smooth, gag reflex intact	Hoarseness; soft palate fails to rise or uvula deviates laterally.
• CN X: symmetry of uvula movement	Symmetrical rising of soft palate	
• CN XI: neck and shoulder strength	Symmetrical strength of trapezii and sternocleid omastoid muscles	Weakness, unilateral or bilateral

Steps	Normal and/or Common Findings	Significant Deviations
• CN XII: tongue control, symmetry, strength	Even strength and motion of tongue	Fasciculations or deviation of tongue

PEDIATRIC ADAPTATIONS

Infant

Steps	Normal and/or Common Findings	Significant Deviations
Inspection		
• Behavior. Note alertness, positioning.	Irritability	Extreme irritability, tremors Brudzinski's or Kernig's sign
• Crying. Note pitch of cry.		High-pitched or cat's cry
• Reflexes. Moro, tonic neck, palmar and plantar grasp, Babinski, rooting, sucking	All present in term newborn	Absence of reflexes
• Neck righting	4–6 months old	
• Parachute	8–9 months old	
• Muscle tone	Firm recoil	Flaccid
• Observe for appropriate parent–infant interactions, stranger anxiety, parent's ability to soothe infant	Separation anxiety greatest at 8–20 months	Inappropriate interactions and parental expectations; no separation anxiety
Palpation		
• Anterior and posterior fontanels	Soft and flat	Bulging or markedly depressed

Continued

TABLE 5 CRANIAL NERVE FUNCTIONS AND ASSESSMENT METHODS

Cranial Nerve	Name	Type	Function	Assessment Methods
I	Olfactory	Sensory	Smell	Ask client to close eyes and identify different mild aromas, such as coffee, tobacco, vanilla, oil of cloves, peanut butter, orange, lemon, lime, chocolate.
II	Optic	Sensory	Vision and visual fields	Ask client to read Snellen chart; check visual fields to confrontation; and conduct an ophthalmoscopic examination.
III	Oculomotor	Motor	Extraocular eye movement (EOM); movement of sphincter of pupil; movement of ciliary muscles of lens	Assess six ocular movements and pupil reaction.
IV	Trochlear	Motor	EOM, specifically moves eyeball downward and laterally	Assess six ocular movements.
V	Trigeminal Ophthalmic branch	Sensory	Sensation of cornea, skin of face, and nasal mucosa	While client looks upward, lightly touch lateral sclera of eye to elicit blink reflex; to test light sensation,

				have client close eyes, wipe a wisp of cotton over client's forehead and paranasal sinuses; to test deep sensation, use alternating blunt and sharp ends of a safety pin over same areas.
	Maxillary branch	Sensory	Sensation of skin of face and anterior oral cavity (tongue and teeth)	Assess skin sensation as for ophthalmic branch above.
	Mandibular branch	Motor and sensory	Muscles of mastication; sensation of skin of face	Ask client to clench teeth.
VI	Abducens	Motor	EOM; moves eyeball laterally	Assess directions of gaze.
VII	Facial	Motor and sensory	Facial expression; taste (anterior two thirds of tongue)	Ask client to smile, raise the eyebrows, frown, puff out cheeks, close eyes tightly; ask client to identify various tastes placed on tip and sides of tongue: sugar (sweet), salt, lemon juice (sour), and quinine (bitter); identify areas of taste.
VIII	Auditory Vestibular branch	Sensory	Equilibrium	Assessment methods are discussed with cerebellar functions (in next section).

155

TABLE 5 CRANIAL NERVE FUNCTIONS AND ASSESSMENT METHODS (Continued)

Cranial Nerve	Name	Type	Function	Assessment Methods
	Cochlear branch	Sensory	Hearing	Assess client's ability to hear spoken word and vibrations of tuning fork.
IX	Glossopharyngeal	Motor and sensory	Swallowing ability and gag reflex, tongue movement, taste (posterior tongue)	Use tongue blade on posterior tongue while client says "ah" to elicit gag reflex; apply tastes on posterior tongue for identification; ask client to move tongue from side to side and up and down.
X	Vagus	Motor and sensory	Sensation of pharynx and larynx; swallowing; vocal cord movement	Assessed with cranial nerve IX; assess client's speech for hoarseness.
XI	Accessory	Motor	Head movement; shrugging of shoulders	Ask client to shrug shoulders against resistance from your hands and turn head to side against resistance from your hand (repeat for other side).
XII	Hypoglossal	Motor	Protusion of tongue	Ask client to protrude tongue at midline, then move it side to side.

Source: From Kozier, B., Erb, G., and Olivieri, R. (1991): *Fundamentals of Nursing*, ed. 4. Addison-Wesley, Reading, MA, Benjamin-Cummings Publishing Company, p. 430, with permission.

Steps	Normal and/or Common Findings	Significant Deviations
• Touch. Note response to touch in extremities in quiet-alert state.	Moves to touch	No response; exaggerated, jerky response; asymmetrical response
Test		
• Hearing. Note acoustic activity.	Responds by waking, or turning toward sound, or movement	No response to sounds
• Pupils	PERRLA	Unequal pupillary response

Child

Steps	Normal and/or Common Findings	Significant Deviations
Inspection		
• Observe for appropriate parent–child interaction	Increasing independence of child, decreasing control by parent	Communication unclear; hostility; aggression; dependence
• Cerebral dominance. Observe child while at play.	Preference for one hand or the other usually evident by age 3–4	
Test		
• Speech	Three-year-olds should be able to speak so that others can understand them 90% of the time.	Unclear speech

Continued

Steps	Normal and/or Common Findings	Significant Deviations
Infant		
• CN II, III, IV, VI	Infant should blink when light is shined in eyes, gaze at close face, track bright object.	Absent, asymmetrical, or diminished response for each area tested
• CN V	Rooting and sucking reflex present.	
• CN VII	Facial symmetry when crying, sucking, and rooting	
• CN VIII	Blink or Moro reflex in response to clapping near side of head	
• CN I and XI: cannot be tested in the infant		
• CN IX and X: similar to the adult		
Child		
• CN II: Snellen eye chart with pictures or E chart may be used.		
• CN III, IV, VI: use a new toy to test cardinal positions.		
• CN V: may offer child a cracker to test muscular strength of jaw		
• Remaining CN may be tested as for an adult.		

Steps	Normal and/or Common Findings	Significant Deviations
• Children who are 3–6 years old should be evaluated by the DDST (Denver Developmental Screening Test)		Abnormal results on the DDST

GERIATRIC ADAPTATIONS

Steps	Normal and/or Common Findings	Significant Deviations
Inspection		
• Face		Tremors, asymmetry such as drooping of side of mouth, drooling from one side of mouth, asymmetrical wrinkling of forehead
• Extremities		Tremors, unilateral or symmetrical weakness, gait disturbances
• Emotional responses		Labile, severely agitated, major behavioral changes
Test		
• Mental acuity. Note alterations.	Diminished memory for recent events	Forgets address or names of close family members
• Heel-to-shin movement	May not be able to perform	

Continued

Steps	Normal and/or Common Findings	Significant Deviations
• Equilibrium *Note:* Do not ask geriatric clients to perform deep knee bends or hop in place on one foot. Most normal elderly people cannot do these maneuvers because of impaired position sense. Instead, observe client rising from chair.	Diminished. Decreased vibratory sense in toes	
Percussion		
• Deep tendon reflexes	May be diminished, especially the Achilles reflex	
Cranial Nerves		
• CN I	Sense of smell diminished	See significant deviations for the adult. Sense of smell absent
• CN II	Diminished peripheral vision, presbyopia corrected with glasses, diminished color discrimination (especially blues, greens, and purples)	Marked loss of vision
• CN III	Pupil size diminished, impaired accommodation, diminished upward gaze	

Steps	Normal and/or Common Findings	Significant Deviations
• CN V	Sensory perception of pain, light touch may be diminished.	
• CN VII	Diminished sense of taste	
• CN VIII	Diminished hearing, especially of high-frequency sounds	
• CN IX and X	Diminished taste perception on posterior tongue	
• CN XI	Diminished muscle strength	

DIAGNOSTIC TESTS

May need to refer for:
- CT scan
- MRI
- EEG
- Electrolytes
- Spinal tap

POSSIBLE NURSING DIAGNOSES

- Communication, impaired verbal
- Coping, ineffective individual
- Physical mobility, impaired
- Swallowing, impaired
- Sensory-perceptual alterations
- Thought processes, altered
- Injury, high risk for

CLINICAL ALERT

• Differentiate symptoms of dementia and delirium and refer all behavioral problems for diagnosis and treatment

SAMPLE DOCUMENTATION

Gait, coordination smooth and steady. Extremities symmetrically strong; touch and vibratory sense intact. DTRs symmetrically + 2 (biceps, triceps, brachioradialis, knee jerk, ankle). Oriented × 3; thought, emotion grossly appropriate. Cranial nerves I–XII intact.

PATIENT/FAMILY EDUCATION AND HOME HEALTH NOTES

Adult

• Prevent head injury with seat belts, helmets.
• Prevent motor vehicle accidents—observe speed limits, do not drink and drive.
• Read labels of pesticides, chemicals and observe precautions.

Pediatric

• Protect infants and toddlers from traumatic falls.
• Teach parents and children use of seat belts, helmets, car seats.
• Teach sports/recreation safety (e.g., spotters for gymnastics; never swim alone, never dive in unknown waters; observe cautions on toys, including age appropriateness).
• Prevent ingestion of poisons, drugs, chemicals. Store all such products out of sight and reach, behind locked door if possible.
• Keep syrup of ipecac on hand. Post poison control number on telephone.

Geriatric

- Maintain activities that stimulate the mind.
- Have assessment and treatment of diminished vision, hearing.
- Maintain physical activities and exercise.
- Take care to avoid extreme heat and cold.

Male Genitalia and Rectum

HISTORY

Adult

- Client's age
- Frequency, urgency, dysuria, nocturia
- Difficulty starting or stopping urinary stream
- Dribbling or weak stream
- Blood in urine; discharge
- Pain, lesions or masses on penis, scrotum, inguinal area, anus
- Circumcised
- Contraceptive use
- Swelling of scrotum
- History of prostatitis, UTIs, pyelonephritis
- History of surgery, trauma
- Satisfied with sexual activity
- Impotence, difficulty getting or maintaining erection
- Sexually transmitted diseases
- Sexual partner preference
- Risk factors for AIDS
- Hemorrhoids
- Rectal bleeding, blood in stools

Pediatric

- Number of wet diapers per day
- Perianal itching
- Meconium ileus
- Chronic constipation, diarrhea, mucorrhea
- Enuresis
- Encopresis
- UTIs
- Scrotal swelling
- Mother's use of hormones during pregnancy
- Sexual activity (adolescent)

Geriatric

- Inability to control urine
- Up at night to void (number of times)
- Retention or incomplete emptying; straining to void
- Hesitancy
- Any treatment or surgery of prostatic enlargement; surgery for hernia
- Decline in frequency of or satisfaction from sexual activity
- Impotence
- Difficulty retracting foreskin

EQUIPMENT

- Gloves
- Lubricant
- Thermometer (for neonates)

PATIENT PREPARATION

- Supine
- Standing
- Bending over

PHYSICAL ASSESSMENT

Steps	Normal and/or Common Findings	Significant Deviations
Inspection		
• Hair. Note distribution, foreign bodies.	Parasites	
• Skin of penis, scrotum, inguinal area	Intact, smooth, wrinkled, rugae on scrotum	Lesions, rashes, nodules, edema, body lice
• Penis. Note preprice, glans, foreskin, circumcision, position of urinary meatus. (See Table 6.)	No lesions, discharge Foreskin easily retracted, if present Located at tip	Phimosis, chancre, warts, ulcers, discharge Displacement on dorsal or ventral side of penis
• Anus	Hemorrhoids (Fig. 49)	Lesions, polyps, bleeding
Palpation Use gloves.		
• Shaft of penis	Slightly tender	Very tender or painful Discharge from urinary meatus; nodules, masses, lesions
• Testicles. Note size.	Smooth, one side usually larger than other, left side lower than right, freely moveable	Tenderness, nodules, ulcers, lesions, pain, enlarged
• Inguinal, femoral areas	No masses, nodes	Hernias, enlarged nodes
• Anus and rectum	Hemorrhoids	Inflammation, rashes, lesions, tenderness, induration Masses

Continued

TABLE 6
**STAGES OF SECONDARY SEXUAL CHARACTERISTICS,
MALE GENITAL DEVELOPMENT**

Development	Characteristic
A. Hair growth	1. None
	2. Scant fine hair at the base of the penis
	3. Darker and curlier hair
	4. Adult type but less hair
	5. Adult
B. Genital development	1. No change
	2. Larger scrotum and testes, skin redder
	3. Enlargement of penis
	4. Further enlargement of penis, scrotal skin thickening
	5. Adult

Source: Adapted from Tanner, J. M.: *Growth at Adolescence,* ed. 2. Blackwell Scientific Publications, Oxford, England, 1962.

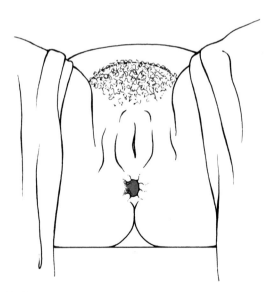

FIGURE 49.
External hemorrhoid.

Steps	Normal and/or Common Findings	Significant Deviations
• Prostate. With client leaning over table, gently insert gloved, lubricated index finger into rectum. Note size, consistency.	Smooth, rubbery; should only be able to palpate about 1 cm of gland; soft	Tenderness, nodules, masses; > 1 cm protruding into rectum; firm, hard

PEDIATRIC ADAPTATIONS

Infant

Steps	Normal and/or Common Findings	Significant Deviations
Inspection		
• Penis. Note preputce and glans.	Smooth, nontender, moist. Prepuce covers glans.	Redness, tenderness, swelling
• Urethral meatus. Note placement. Retract foreskin in uncircumsized males only enough to see urinary meatus. Do not break adhesions.	Centered at tip of penis	Hypospadias, meatus on dorsal or ventral side Epispadias
• Scrotum	Well rugated, both palpable, nontender	Absence of rugae or underdeveloped scrotum
• Testes		Either or both absent
• Rectal opening	Patent	Absent, occluded
• Meconium	Should pass within 24 hours of birth	Meconium ileus

Continued

Steps	Normal and/or Common Findings	Significant Deviations
Palpation		
• Testicles. To check for their presence in scrotum, position child cross-legged and sitting to prevent retraction of testes.	Both palpable	Either or both absent
• Inguinal canal	Intact	Herniations, bulges
• Test: If perianal itching, place tape against perianal folds. Examine with microscope.	No nematodes visible	Nematodes
• Test: Anal patency can be checked in neonates by cautiously inserting a lubricated rectal thermometer if stools are not passed within first 24 hours of life.	Anus patent	Unable to insert thermometer

GERIATRIC ADAPTATIONS

Steps	Normal and/or Common Findings	Significant Deviations
Inspection		
• Pubic hair. Note amount and distribution.	Diminished if not absent	

Steps	Normal and/or Common Findings	Significant Deviations
• Penis. Retract foreskin, if present, to examine head of penis. Note hygiene.	Decrease in size Many men > age 75 have not been circumcised.	Drainage, infection, lesions, nodules, tenderness
• Scrotum	Pendulous	
Palpation		
• Testes. Note size.	Small, atrophied	Nodules
• Rectum	Enlarged prostate, relaxed rectal sphincter tone	Polyps, bleeding Fecal impaction

DIAGNOSTIC TESTS

May need to refer for:
- Culture, if drainage is present
- Fecal swab for guaiac test
- Urinalysis

POSSIBLE NURSING DIAGNOSES

- Infection, high risk for
- Constipation
- Nutrition, altered
- Fluid volume deficit, regulatory failure
- Urinary elimination, altered patterns of
- Urinary retention
- Sexual dysfunction
- Altered sexuality patterns
- Self-care deficit: bathing/hygiene
- Self-care deficit: toileting
- Rape-trauma syndrome

CLINICAL ALERT

- Maintain client's privacy and reduce embarrassment as much as possible.
- Prevent trauma to hemorrhoids.

SAMPLE DOCUMENTATION

Skin of genitalia smooth, dry, nontender. Circumcised penis without discharge or lesions. Testes smooth, not enlarged. No hernias palpated. Prostate border palpable; smooth, firm, nontender.

PATIENT/FAMILY EDUCATION AND HOME HEALTH NOTES

Adult

- Instruct men in TSE beginning in midteens.
- Explain prevention of sexually transmitted diseases by limiting activity to one, mutually monogamous, uninfected partner; if not possible, use condom with every exposure: emphasize risk of multiple partners.
- Rectal exam annually after age 40.

Pediatric

- Discuss testicular exams.
- Discuss sexual development and activities as appropriate for age.
- Teach parents/child how to keep uncircumcised penis clean.

Geriatric

- Encourage intake of 2,000 to 3,000 ml of fluid daily.
- Avoid micturition syncope in bathroom possibly resulting in a serious fall (teach client to sit down to void).

- If not circumcised, keep head of penis clean.
- Use water-soluble lubricant if needed during intercourse.

Female Genitalia and Rectum

HISTORY

Adult

- Menstrual history
  - Age at menarche
  - LMP
  - Character, length, regularity of menses
  - Dysmenorrhea: nature, severity, treatment
  - Premenstrual changes: nature, severity, treatment
- Sexual history
  - Age at onset
  - Number of different partners
  - Sexual partner preference
  - Satisfactions, problems
- Contraceptive history
  - Current and previous methods used
  - Current method: satisfaction, consistency, questions or problems noted
- Obstetric history
  - Gravidity, parity (term, preterm, living children)
  - Abortions (spontaneous, induced)
  - Previous pregnancies: complications with pregnancy, delivery, newborn
- Use of these products: douche, sprays, deodorants, antiseptic soaps
- Dates of last Pap smear and pelvic examination
- History of vaginitis, cystitis, pyelonephritis, in utero exposure to DES, sexually transmitted diseases
- Recent change in any of the following: bleeding, pain, vaginal discharge, urinary frequency or dysuria

- History of gynecologic surgeries
- History of sexual assault, incest; stage in crisis resolution
- Risk factors for AIDS

Pediatric

- Hygienic practices:
  - Use of bubble baths, irritating soaps, powders
  - Number of layers of clothing
  - Wearing cotton underpants
  - Cleansing perineal area front-to-back
- Signs of sexual abuse: trauma; skin color changes in perianal area; history of bleeding, itching; inappropriate adultlike sexual knowledge, language, behavior

Geriatric

- Menopausal history (date, difficulties, satisfactions)
- Soreness, tenderness of vaginal wall
- Dyspareunia
- Pressure or heavy sensation in genital area
- Involuntary urination with laugh, cough, sneeze
- Vaginal bleeding since menopause
- Adaptations in sexual activity

EQUIPMENT

- Gown, drape
- Sterile glove
- Lubricant
- Flexible floor lamp
- Pap smear equipment
- Speculum (may need pediatric size for both young women and older women who are no longer sexually active)

PATIENT PREPARATION

- Have client empty bladder before examination.
- Drape fully in lithotomy position.

- Offer mirror to explain findings to client.
- Warm speculum to body temperature.

PHYSICAL ASSESSMENT—EXTERNAL STRUCTURES

Steps	Normal and/or Common Findings	Significant Deviations
Inspection		
• Hair. Note distribution, amount, foreign bodies.	Coarse, full, symmetrical	Uneven or unusually sparse Lice
• Labia. Note color, vascularity, moisture, symmetry, discharge, lesions, odor.	Pink to red. Moist, symmetrical Scant to moderate white, nonodorous discharge	Pale, inflamed Varicosities Dry Edema or swelling, especialy unilaterally Dry, caked discharge Copius, watery, thickened, or foul-smelling, white-yellow or green discharge, lesions
• Clitoris. Note size, color, lesions.	2×0.5 cm, same color as surrounding tissue	Atrophied or enlarged; reddened
• Vaginal and urinary orifices. Note color, lesions, moisture, size, bulging of vaginal wall.	Pink to red, moist, smooth. No lesions bulging	Reddened; lesions (ulcers, blisters, condyloma accuminata), edematous, irritated Bulging of anterior or posterior vaginal wall on straining
• Anus. Note integrity.	Wrinkled, coarsened texture	Fissures, hemorrhoids, lesions

Continued

Steps	Normal and/or Common Findings	Significant Deviations
Palpation		
• Labia. Note masses, tenderness, integrity.	Smooth, nontender, homogenous tissue	Nodules, painful to touch, irregularities
• Skene glands. Use one finger to press upward and laterally inside vagina, drawing finger toward outside of vagina. observe for drainage from gland.	No discharge Openings not visible	Discharge (culture) Openings visible
• Bartholin glands	No tenderness or edema	Redness, tenderness, swelling of labia, especially unilaterally
• Vaginal orifices. Use thumb and forefinger; gently pinch around sides and perineal area. Note tenderness, masses.	No masses, nontender	Nodules, painful to touch
• With finger in vagina, ask client to tighten muscles and bear down. Note strength, bulges, urinary incontinence.	Tight muscles, no bulges, no incontinence	Bulging of anterior or posterior wall, urinary incontinence, protrusion of cervix

PHYSICAL ASSESSMENT—INTERNAL STRUCTURES

To insert vaginal speculum: Warm speculum with water. Insert two fingers into vagina and press down firmly; insert closed speculum at an angle over fingers, keeping blades at 45° downward angle. Rotate speculum back to horizontal level and gently open blades.

Steps	Normal and/or Common Findings	Significant Deviations
Inspection		
• Mucosa. Note color, integrity, lesions, discharge.	Pink to red; smooth, moist, clear to white odorless discharge	Bright red or pale; lesions, fissures, inflamed areas, discharge
• Cervix. Note color, position, surface, discharge, os, lesions.	Evenly pink, midline, smooth surface or small, raised, light nabothian cysts. Discharge odorless, clear to white. Os small, round or horizontal slit	Blue, reddened, pale Deviated laterally Patches of red or white tissue, friability increased Heavy, malodorous, yellow to green to gray discharge

OBTAINING PAP SMEARS

With speculum in place, obtain cells from cervical os, cervical border, and vaginal pool. Use either spatula or brushes, and label slides as *ectocervical* or *endocervical* after spraying with fixative. (To withdraw speculum: Close blades, rotate 45°, gently remove, avoid pinching.)

Steps	Normal and/or Common Findings	Significant Deviations
Palpation		
Insert gloved index and middle fingers into vagina and place nondominant hand on lower abdomen. Trap internal structures between your hands.		
• Cervix. Note consistency, surface, position, mobility, tenderness, patency of os.	Firm, smooth, midline, mobile to 2 cm, nontender, patent	Boggy, nodules, lateral deviations, fixed, painful with movement, strictures at os

Continued

Steps	Normal and/or Common Findings	Significant Deviations
• Uterus. Note position, size, shape, mobility, tenderness, masses.	Midline. Pear-shaped, 6–8 cm in length, slight AP mobility without tenderness	Lateral deviation, unilateral or bilateral masses, fixed, tender or painful to touch
• Ovaries. Note size, shape, tenderness, consistency, masses.	May not be palpable. Approximately 3 × 2 cm, slightly tender, smooth, firm	Enlarged, nodular, asymmetrical, painful

Change gloves. Lubricate. Insert index finger into vagina, middle finger into rectum.

• Uterus. Note shape, masses.	Smooth, uniform, no masses	Masses, irregular shape
• Rectal wall. Note masses, tenderness, tone.	Smooth, nontender, firm muscle tone	Nodules, masses, lesions
		Tender
(Obtain stool specium from gloved hand)		Absent tone

PEDIATRIC ADAPTATIONS

Infant

Steps	Norman/Common Findings	Significant Deviations
Inspection		
• Discharge. Note presence.	Absent or slight white discharge or blood in first week	
• Labia. Note size, position.	Edematous, slightly opened	Ambiguous genitalia
• Vaginal opening. Note presence.	Patent	Absence of vaginal opening
• Rectum	Meconium passed in 24 hours	No meconium in 24 hours

Child

Steps	Normal/Common Findings	Significant Deviations
Inspection		
Note: complete gyne-cological exams, including Pap smear, should begin when individual becomes sexually active or at age 18–20.		
• Hair growth.	No hair—preadoles-cent	
	Slight fine hair on labia majora—hair darker, thicker but finer texture and amount less than adult	
• Genital region. Note signs of sex-ual abuse.	No signs of abuse Hymenal tag	Scarring, lesions, red or darkened pig-ment, poor sphinc-ter tone, vaginal odor (and other signs of infection), bleeding, pain, presence of STDs

GERIATRIC ADAPTATIONS

Steps	Normal/Common Findings	Significant Deviations
Inspection		
• External genitalia	Atrophied. Dimin-ished fat pads. Sparse, white hair	Masses

Continued

Steps	Normal and/or Common Findings	Significant Deviations
• Mucosa	Pale, thin, friable	Tears, lesions, erythematous
• Secretions, discharges	Scanty to absent	Colored, malodorous, or abundant discharges
• Uterus, ovaries	Nontender, atrophied, smaller. Ovaries should not be palpable.	Pain, asymmetry, enlarged

DIAGNOSTIC TESTS

May need to refer for:
- Pap smear
- Other smears and cultures: gonococcal culture, chlamydial enzyme immunoassay, wet and dry mounts for other microbes
- Guaiac test of stool

POSSIBLE NURSING DIAGNOSES

- Pain acute
- Rape-trauma syndrome
- Self-care deficit: bathing/hygiene
- Sexual dysfunction
- Sexuality patterns, altered

CLINICAL ALERT

- Signs of sexual assault
- Masses
- Unusual pain
- Postmenopausal bleeding
- Infection signs and symptoms
- Pregnancy signs

SAMPLE DOCUMENTATION

External genitalia nontender, not inflamed; normal hair distribution. Vaginal mucosa pink, moist, smooth. Cervix nulliparous, pink, without ulcers or nodules. Pap smear obtained. Uterus palpable, nonpregnant size, without masses or tenderness. Ovaries nontender. Rectum without hemorrhoids, masses, tenderness. Rectal wall smooth, firm, nontender.

PATIENT EDUCATION/HOME HEALTH NOTES

Adult

- Teach good hygiene and prevention of cystitis/vaginitis:
  - Cleanse front to back.
  - Wear loose clothing, as few layers as possible.
  - Wear cotton underpants; avoid pantyhose when possible.
  - Urinate after intercourse.
  - Avoid tub baths, bubble bath, strongly perfumed soaps and powders.
  - Never use vaginal deodorants, deodorized tampons or pads.
  - Avoid vaginal douches.
  - Drink more fluids ($>$ 8 glasses/day) if a history of cystitis
- Pap smear schedule: after two normal smears, repeat every 2–3 years until age 40 if not at high risk (multiple partners, early onset of sexual activity, family history of cancer). Every year after age 40.
- Teach about contraception.
- Teach prevention of STD by limiting activity to one mutually monogamous, uninfected partner; use condom with every exposure; emphasize risk of multiple partners (both STD and cervical cancer).

Pediatric

- Teach good hygiene as outlined above.
- Teach about contraception and STD prevention as indicated by age and sexual activity.
- Teach parents/child techniques in self-protection; for exam-

ple, *always* tell parent or another adult if touched, threatened, hurt; assertively refuse to be touched, touch, look at, or show intimate parts; sexual assault is the fault of the adult, not the child.

Geriatric

- Teach about normal changes associated with aging; for example, need for water-soluble lubricant for intercourse.
- Sexual activity is normal into the 80s and 90s if there are no major health problems and an acceptable partner is available.
- Continue pelvic exam by health care professional annually and Pap smear as indicated.

PREGNANCY

HISTORY

Adult

Antepartum

Ask about the following:
- Age
- LMP
- Menstrual history (see Reproductive)
- Contraceptive history (see Reproductive)
- Gravidity, parity, number of preterm births
- Number of abortions, spontaneous or induced, and gestation of each
- Number of living children
- Previous obstetrical history
- Health since LMP; if illnesses, nature and treatment
- Accident/trauma history since pregnancy or with prior pregnancies. If significant, explore possibility of battering.
- Use of tobacco, alcohol, any drugs since LMP: note amount, frequency.
- Cat in home

- Know genetic/chromosomal abnormalities of either parent or family
- Months attempted conception
- Weight at LMP
- Dietary pattern
- Date of quickening
- Problems with this pregnancy
- Daily routine
- Knowledge of pregnancy and normal changes
- Relationships with father of baby and other family; degree of perceived support

Postpartum

- Note delivery date, length of labor, route of delivery, complications, status of infant.
- Breast or bottle feeding
- Adequacy or difficulty in self-care (specify)
- Adequacy or difficulty in newborn care: feeding, bathing, dressing, comforting
- Ability of support person to assist in care of mother and infant
- Contraception planned

EQUIPMENT

- Stethoscope
- Sphygomanometer
- Centimeter tape
- Fetoscope
- Speculum
- Glove
- Urinalysis for glucose, protein

PATIENT PREPARATION

- Sitting and lying positions
- Have client empty bladder, obtain urine specimen (clean).
- Have client in supine position as little as possible.

PHYSICAL ASSESSMENT

Steps	Normal and/or Common Findings	Significant Deviations
	ANTEPARTUM	

Inspection

Steps	Normal and/or Common Findings	Significant Deviations
• Face and head. Note color, pigmentation, edema.	Chloasma, no edema, nasal stuffiness	Edema, especially periorbital and around bridge of nose
• Breasts. Note size, vascularity, color.	Increased size, visible vessels symmetrically, darkened areolar areas	Pain, redness, warmth
• Abdomen. Note size, shape, color striae, umbilical flattening.	Size (see Fig. 50); ovoid shape, striae, linea nigra may be present, umbilicus flattens after 30 weeks.	Size not appropriate to gestational age
• Cervix. Note color, shape, of os, discharge.	Dark pink to blue (at 8–12 weeks); softened; os close in nulliparas, slitlike opening in multiparas; no bleeding, increased white creamy discharge	Frank bleeding not associated with examination or intercourse
• Musculoskeletal	Increased lumbar curve and waddling gait in last trimester; mild dependent edema with prolonged standing	Marked dependent edema

Palpation

Steps	Normal and/or Common Findings	Significant Deviations
• Abdomen. Note size, pain.	Fundal height palpable after 12–13 weeks (see Fig. 50)	Fundal height not appropriate to gestational age; painful to palpate

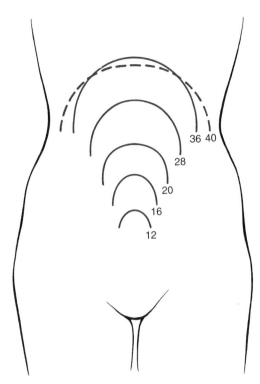

FIGURE 50.
Fundal heights and gestation.

Steps	Normal and/or Common Findings	Significant Deviations
• Neurologic. Note reflex irritability.	Reflexes +2 No clonus	Reflexes +3 or +4; clonus of ankle
Auscultation • Heart. Note rate, other sounds. Note blood pressure.	Rate may increase 10–15 beats per minute. May have short systolic murmurs	Tachycardia; marked murmurs, palpitations

Continued

Steps	Normal and/or Common Findings	Significant Deviations
ANTEPARTUM (*continued*)		
• Blood pressure	First and third trimesters at prepregnant level; falls in second trimester	> 140/90 or systolic increase of 30 mm Hg; diastolic increase of 15 mm Hg (if elevated, turn to left side; test urine for protein)
• Fetal heart. Note rate, rhythm, location (on mother's abdomen as RUQ, RLQ, LUQ, RUQ).	> 160 at 12 weeks decreasing to 110–160 in late pregnancy; increases 15 beats per minute with activity; regular or slightly irregular rhythm	Not audible after 12 weeks with Doppler; not audible after 18–20 weeks with fetoscope. Rate < 110–120 in last trimester; no increase in rate with fetal movement; pattern of irregularity
POSTPARTUM		

Inspection

• Breasts. Note color, feeding ability.	No redness. Infant able to root, grasp areolar tissue in mouth, suck 5 minutes each side first days in at least two positions	Redness. Infant unable to suck 5 minutes each side
• Abdomen. Note uterine, bladder positions.	Not visible or midline, below umbilicus	Easily visible above umbilicus or deviated laterally
• Perineum. Note color, integrity, swelling, drainage.	Slight redness, mild edema, lochia appropriate to time (rubra to serosa)	Bright red or unilateral redness; continued lochia rubra beyond first

Steps	Normal and/or Common Findings	Significant Deviations
	If episiotomy, no signs of infection of incision	days; bright red bleeding; signs of infection of episiotomy
	If hemorrhoids, may be swollen	
Palpation		
• Breast. Wash hands before touching. Note warmth, hard areas, tenderness or pain.	Mild uniform warmth, no masses, some tenderness, especially nipples	Hot areas, hardened areas, painful to touch
• Abdomen. Note fundal height, firmness; bladder, tenderness.	Day 1: at umbilicus, firm	Fundus boggy, elevated, deviated laterally; bladder palpable with suprapubic tenderness
	Day 2: umbilicus + 1–2 cm	
	Day 3: at umbilicus	
	Day 4: steady decrease	
	Bladder not palpable	
• Legs. Gently palpate calves for heat, tenderness. Dorsiflex ankle and ask client if pain felt in calf.	No heat	Heat, pain on dorsiflexion (positive Homan's sign)
	No pain (negative Homan's sign)	
• Skin. Note temperature, moisture.	Warm (oral temperature < 100.4°F); increased perspiration	Temperature > 100.4°F

DIAGNOSTIC TESTS

May need to refer for:
• CBC
• UA
• Ultrasonography
• Pelvimetry

POSSIBLE NURSING DIAGNOSES

- Sleep pattern disturbance
- Breastfeeding, effective, ineffective
- Knowledge deficit [learning need]
- Fatigue
- Growth and development, altered
- Body image disturbance
- Nutrition, altered: more or less than body requirements
- Family processes, altered

CLINICAL ALERT

- Elevated blood pressure, facial edema, proteinuria, glucosuria, headache
- Fetal heart rate abnormalities
- Uterine growth disproportionate to gestational age
- Mother's report of decreased fetal movement
- Bleeding not associated with examination or intercourse
- Abdominal pain

SAMPLE DOCUMENTATION

Age 33; G ii, Pi, LCi, Abo. Approximately 22 weeks gestation (LMP 5/26; EDC 2/28). Fundus at umbilicus, FHT 170 LLQ. Urine neg/neg; weight 158; BP 100/70. No bleeding, headache, pain reported. Vaginal examination: cervix closed, soft, thick.

PATIENT/FAMILY EDUCATION AND HOME HEALTH NOTES

- Teach normal changes of pregnancy, maternal and fetal development.
- Review dietary needs every month. Assess with recall if weight gain too much or too little.
- Encourage in moderate exercise (e.g., walking, swimming) and rest.

- Teach danger signs in pregnancy.
- Teach warning signs of labor.
- Teach infant care, normal growth and development.
- Discuss breastfeeding, provide information and support.

Nursing Diagnoses

NORTH AMERICAN NURSING DIAGNOSIS ASSOCIATION (NANDA) 1992 APPROVED NURSING DIAGNOSTIC CATEGORIES:

Activity intolerance
Activity intolerance, high risk for
Adjustment, impaired
Airway clearance, ineffective
Anxiety
Aspiration, high risk for
Body image disturbance
Body temperature, altered, high risk for
Bowel incontinence
Breastfeeding, effective
Breastfeeding, ineffective
Breastfeeding, interrupted
Breathing pattern, ineffective
Cardiac output, decreased
Communication, impaired verbal
Constipation
Constipation, colonic
Constipation, perceived
Coping, defensive
Coping, ineffective individual
Decisional conflict (specify)
Denial, ineffective
Diarrhea
Disuse syndrome, high risk for

Diversional activity deficit
Dysreflexia
Family coping, compromised
Family coping, disabling
Family coping, potential for growth
Family processes, altered
Fatigue
Fear
Fluid volume deficit
Fluid volume deficit, high risk for
Fluid volume excess
Gas exchange, impaired
Grieving, anticipatory
Grieving, dysfunctional
Growth and development, altered
Health maintenance, altered
Health-seeking behaviors (specify)
Home maintenance management, impaired
Hopelessness
Hyperthermia
Hypothermia
Incontinence, functional

NORTH AMERICAN NURSING DIAGNOSIS ASSOCIATION (NANDA) 1992 APPROVED NURSING DIAGNOSTIC CATEGORIES (*Continued*)

Incontinence, reflex
Incontinence, stress
Incontinence, total
Incontinence, urge
Infection, high risk for
Injury, high risk for
Knowledge deficit (specify)
Noncompliance (specify)
Nutrition, altered: less than body requirements
Nutrition, altered: more than body requirements
Nutrition, altered: high risk for more than body requirements
Oral mucous membrane, altered
Pain [acute]
Pain, chronic
Parental role conflict
Parenting, altered
Parenting, altered, high risk for
Personal identity disturbance
Physical mobility, impaired
Poisoning, high risk for
Post-trauma response
Powerlessness
Protection, altered
Rape-trauma syndrome
Rape-trauma syndrome: compound reaction
Rape-trauma syndrome: silent reaction
Role performance, altered
Self-care deficit: bathing/hygiene
Self-care deficit: dressing/grooming

Self-care deficit: feeding
Self-care deficit: toileting
Self-esteem disturbance
Self-esteem, chronic low
Self-esteem, situational low
Sensory-perceptual alterations: visual, auditory, kinesthetic, gustatory, tactile, olfactory (specify)
Sexual dysfunction
Sexuality patterns, altered
Skin integrity, impaired
Skin integrity, impaired, high risk for
Sleep pattern disturbance
Social interaction, impaired
Social isolation
Spiritual distress
Suffocation, high risk for
Swallowing, impaired
Thermoregulation, ineffective
Thought processes, altered
Tissue integrity, impaired
Tissue perfusion, altered: cerebral, cardiopulmonary, gastrointestinal, peripheral (specify type), renal
Trauma, high risk for
Unilateral neglect
Urinary elimination, altered patterns of
Urinary retention [acute/chronic]
Violence, Potential: Self-directed or directed at others

From *North American Nursing Diagnosis Association Guidelines* (1992). Taxonomy 1-revised. NANDA, St. Louis, with permission.

Sample Nursing History Form

Date _____ Name _____

Room _____ Sex: M   F

Address _____

Telephone Number _____

Private Home _____ Apartment _____

Retirement center _____ Nursing home _____

Date of birth _____ Age _____

Date of Admission _____ Date of Surg _____

Marital status: M   W   S   D

If widowed, how long? _____

Retired _____ Occupation _____

Social Security number _____

Medicare number _____

Medicaid number _____

Insurance name _____

Number _____

Religious preference: _____

Contact in emergency _____

Reason for seeking care (chief complaint) _____

_____

History of Present Illness/Condition/Surgery

_____

_____

_____

Patient's understanding of current condition: _____

_____

Current diet: _____

Medications currently prescribed: _____

_____

Past Health/Medical History

_____

_____

_____

Allergies (food, medicines, environmental): _____

_____

Medications and treatments at home: _____

_____

Chemical use

Number of cigarettes per day ____   Amount of coffee/tea/
                                        carbonated
Other tobacco per day ____
                                        beverages per day _
Number of years smoked ____
                                        Amount of alcoholic

                                        drinks per day ____

                                        Type _____

Use of other substances _____

_____

Rest and Sleep Patterns

Hours worked per day ____   Rest periods or naps (when,

Hours of sleep per night ____   number, length) _____

Medications used to aid sleep _____

Other measures to aid sleep _____

Sleep problems _____

_____

Mobility and Exercise Patterns:

Type of activity/exercise _____

Amount (times per week: minutes per day) _____

Restrictions/mechanical aids/prostheses/wheel chair/walker/
bedrails

_____

Ability to care for self _____

_____

Diet	*Breakfast*	*Lunch*	*Dinner*	*Snacks*
24-hour recall of previous day				
Usual time of meals at home				

Ability to feed self _____ Dentures _____

Dietary restrictions/dislikes/difficulty _____

Fluid intake per day (type and amount) _____

Elimination (routines, frequency, problems, aids):

Bowel _____

_____

Urinary _____

_____

Communication

Ability to understand English _____

Language spoken _____

Hearing _____ Sight _____ Aids _____

Educational level _____

Ability to speak _____

Orientation Person _____ Time _____

Place _____

Present emotional state _____

Activities

Hobbies _____

Part-time employment _____

Volunteer work _____

Other _____

Family History

Composition
    Number in household
    Roles
Primary support system
History of family health/illness
Other pertinent data

Environmental History

SYSTEM	HISTORY	NOT ASKED
Review of Systems		
General overview		
Skin, hair, nails		
Head and neck		
Eyes		

SYSTEM	HISTORY	NOT ASKED
Review of Systems (*continued*)		
Ears		
Nose/sinus		
Mouth/throat		
Respiratory		
Cardiovascular		
Gastrointestinal		
Breasts/axillae		
Genitourinary		

SYSTEM	HISTORY	NOT ASKED
Musculoskeletal		
Neurologic		
Other pertinent data:		

Adapted from Nursing History Form 584, Harris College of Nursing, Texas Christian University, Fort Worth, TX, with permission.

Sample Physical Assessment Form with Guide

Name _____ Date _____
Age _____ Height _____ Weight _____
Vital Signs: T _____ P _____ R _____
B/P: Sitting _____ Standing _____ Lying _____

EXAMINATION	DESCRIPTION*	NOT EXAMINED
Overall appearance		
Skin		

Adapted from Physical Assessment Form 584. Harris College of Nursing, Texas Christian University, Fort Worth, TX, with permission.

EXAMINATION	DESCRIPTION*	NOT EXAMINED
Head		
Eyes		
Ears		
Nose and sinuses		
Mouth and pharynx		
Neck		
Thorax and lungs		
Breasts and axillae		
Heart and peripheral vascular		

EXAMINATION	DESCRIPTION*	NOT EXAMINED
Abdomen		
Musculoskeletal		
Genitourinary and rectum		
Neurologic		
Mental status		
Laboratory and other pertinent data:		

Physical Assessment Guide

GENERAL INSTRUCTIONS

Use this guide for suggested descriptive terminology for documentation on the Sample Physical Assessment Form.

Be specific, descriptive, and objective. Avoid such terms as "normal," "within normal limits," "good," "fair," "O.K.," and so forth. Describe what you observe rather than making inferences or judgments.

OVERALL APPEARANCE INSPECTION

SEX: male/female

GENERAL GROOMING: clean? hair combed? make-up?

POSITION/POSTURING: supine? prone? rigid? opisthotonos? erect? slumped?

BODY SIZE: thin? fat? obese? emaciated? flabby? weight proportionate to height? mesomorph? endomorph? ectomorph?

FACIAL EXPRESSIONS: smiling? frowning? blank? apathetic?

BODY LANGUAGE: eye contact? no eye contact? arms folded over chest?

OTHER OBSERVATIONS: restless? fidgeting? lying quietly? listless? trembling? tense?

SKIN INSPECTION AND PALPATION

COLOR AND VASCULARITY: pink? tan? brown? dark brown? grayish? pasty? yellowish? flushed? jaundiced?

TURGOR AND MOBILITY: elastic? nonelastic? tenting? wrinkled? edematous? tight?

TEMPERATURE AND MOISTURE: cold? cool? warm? hot? feverish? moist? dry? clammy? oily? sweating? diaphoresis?

TEXTURE: smooth? rough? fine? thick? coarse? scaly? puffy?

NAILS: clean? manicured? smooth? rough? dry? hard? brittle? splitting? cracking? angle of nail bed? clubbing? curved? flat? thick? yellowing? paronychia? *Nail beds and lunule:* pale? pink? cyanotic? red? shape of lunule? blanching? spooning?

BODY HAIR GROWTH: color? thick? thin? coarse? fine? location and distribution on body? hirsutism?

SKIN INTEGRITY: intact? not intact? *Lesions, birthmarks, moles, scars and rashes:* (describe shape, size and location) nevi? fissures? maculas? papules? pustules? nodules? bullae? cysts? carbuncle? wheals? erythema? excoriation? desquamation? abrasions? cherry angiomas? senile lentigines? senile purpura? senile keratoses? seborrheic keratoses? bruises? insect bites? crusts? warts? pimples? blackheads? bleeding? drainage? lacerations? scaly? ulcers? lichenification?

HEAD INSPECTION AND PALPATION

SHAPE: round? oval? square? pointed? normocephalic?

FACE: oval? heart-shaped? pear? long, square? round? thin? high cheekbones? symmetrical?

SENSATION (TRIGEMINAL CN V): sensation on three branches? clenched teeth?

FACIAL CN VII: facial expressions, smiles?

HAIR: Color and growth: coarse? fine? thick? thin? sparse? alopecia? long? short? curly? straight? permed? glossy? shiny? greasy? dry? brittle? stringy? frizzy?

CONDITION OF SCALP: clean? scaly? dandruff? rashes? sores? drainage? *Masses and lumps:* (describe location and shape; measure size.)

EYES INSPECTION AND PALPATION

EYEBROWS: Color and shape: alignment? straight? curved? thick? thin? sparse? plucked? scaly?

EYELASHES: long? short? curved? none? artificial?

EYELIDS: dark? swollen? inflamed? red? stye? infected? open and close simultaneously? ptosis? entropion? ectropion? lid lag? xanthomas?

SHAPE AND APPEARANCE OF EYES: almond? rounded? squinty? prominent? exophthalmic? sunken? symmetrical? bright? clear? dull? tearing? discharge? (serous? purulent?) exotropia? esotropia? nystigmus? strabismus?

SCLERA: white? cream? yellowish? jaundiced? injected? pterygium?

CONJUNCTIVA: pale pink? pink? red? inflamed? nodules? swelling?

IRIS: Color and shape: round? not round? coloboma? arcus senilis?

CORNEA: clear? milky? opaque? cloudy?

PUPILS (OCULOMOTOR—CN III) [PERRLA]: *Size and shape:* (measure in mm) round? not round? (describe) *Equality:* symmetrical? anisocoria? right larger than left? left larger than right? convergence? Reaction to light and accommodation? consensual reaction? EXTRA-OCULAR MOVEMENTS (OCULOMOTOR), TROCHLEAR, ABDUCENS—CN III, IV, VI): intact?

LACRIMAL GLANDS: tender? nontender? inflamed? swollen? tearing?

AIDS: glasses? contact lenses? prosthesis?

VISUAL FIELDS (OPTIC—CN II): intact?

VISION (OPTIC—CN II): reads newsprint? reports objects across room?

EARS INSPECTION AND PALPATION

PINNAE: Size and shape: large? small? in proportion to face? protruding? oval? large lobes? small lobes? symmetrical? right larger than left? left larger than right? pinnae irregular? color? skin intact? redness? swelling? tophi? cauliflower ear? furuncles? Darwin's tubercle?

LEVEL IN RELATION TO EYES: top of pinnae level with outer canthus of eyes? top of pinnae lower than outer canthus of eyes? top of pinnae higher than outer canthus of eyes? *Canal:* clean? discharge? (serous? bloody? purulent?) nodules? inflammation? redness? foreign object? *Cilia:* present/absent? *Cerumen:* present/absent? color? consistency?

TYMPANIC MEMBRANE: color? pearly white? injected? red? inflamed? discharge? cone of light? landmarks? scarring? bubbles? fluid level?

HEARING (AUDITORY—CN VII): right—present/absent? left—present/absent? hears watch tick? hears whisper? responds readily when spoken to? *Weber:* lateralizes equally? to left/right side? *Rinne:* Air conduction > bone conduction 2:1? *Hearing aid:* right/left.

NOSE AND SINUSES INSPECTION AND PALPATION

SIZE AND SHAPE: long? short? large? small? in proportion to face? flat? broad? broad based? thick? thin? enlarged? nares symmetrical/asymmetrical? pointed? swollen? bulbous? flaring of nostrils?

SEPTUM: midline? deviated right/left? perforated?

NASAL MUCOSA AND TURBINATES: pink? pale? bluish? red? dry? moist? discharge? (purulent? clear? watery? mucus?) cilia present/absent? rhinitis? epistaxis? polyps?

PATENCY OF NARES: (close each side and ask client to breathe) right—patent/partial obstruction/obstructed? left—patent/partial obstruction/obstructed?

OLFACTORY (CN I) Correctly identifies odors?

SINUSES: tender? nontender? transillumination?

MOUTH AND PHARYNX INSPECTION

LIPS: *Color:* pink? red? tan? pale? cyanotic? *Shape:* thin? thick? enlarged? swollen? symmetrical/asymmetrical? drooping left side? drooping right side? *Condition:* soft? smooth? dry? cracked? fissured? blisters? lesions? (describe)

TEETH: *Color and condition:* white? yellow? grayish? spotted? stained? darkened? pitting? notched? straight? crooked, protruding? separated? crowded? irregular? broken? notching? peglike? loose? dull? bright? edentulous? malocclusion? *Caries and fillings:* number and location? *Dental hygiene:* clean? not clean?

BREATH ODOR: sweet? odorless? halitosis? musty? acetone? foul? fetid? odor of drugs or food? hot? sour? alcohol?

GUMS: pink? firm? swollen? bleeding? sensitive? gingivitis? hypertrophy? nodules? irritated? receding? moist? ulcerated? dry? shrunken? blistered? spongy?

FACIAL AND GLOSSOPHARYNGEAL (CN VII and IX): identifies taste?

TONGUE: macroglossia? microglossia? glossitis? geographic? red? pink? pale? bluish? brownish? swollen? clean? thin? thick? fissured? raw? coated? moist? dry? cracked? glistening? papillae?

HYPOGLOSSAL (CN XII): *Tongue movement:* symmetry? lateral? fasciculation?

MUCOSA: color? leukoplakia? dry? moist? intact? not intact? masses? (describe size, shape and location) chancre?

PALATE: moist? dry? color? intact? not intact?

UVULA: color? midline? Remains at midline when saying ''ah''? gag reflex present?

PHARYNX: color? petechia? injected? beefy? dysphagia?

TONSILS: present/absent? cryptic? beefy? size 1+ to 4 +?

TEMPOROMANDIBULAR JOINT: fully mobile? symmetrical? tenderness? crepitus?

NECK INSPECTION AND PALPATION

APPEARANCE: long? short? thick? thin? masses? (describe size and shape) symmetrical? not symmetrical?

THYROID: palpable? nodules? tender?

TRACHEA: midline? deviated to right/left?

LYMPH NODES: (occipital, preauricular, postauricular, submental, submaxillary, tonsilar, anterior cervical, posterior cervical, superficial cervical, deep cervical, supraclavicular) nonpalpable? tender? lymphadenopathy? shotty? hard? firm?

THORAX AND LUNGS INSPECTION, PALPATION, PERCUSSION AND AUSCULTATION

RESPIRATIONS: rate? tachypnea, eupnea, bradypnea? apnea? orthopnea? labored? stertorous? *Rhythm:* regular/irregular? inspiration time greater than expiration time? expiration time greater than inspiration time? spasmodic? gasping? orthopnic? gasping? deep? eupnic? shallow? flaring of nostrils with respirations? symmetrical/asymmetrical? right thorax greater than left? left thorax greater than right? ratio of AP diameter to lateral diameter between 1:2 and 5:7? ribs sloped downward at 45° angle? well-defined costal space? accessory muscles used? pigeon chest? funnel chest? barrel chest? abdominal or chest breather? skin intact? lesions? color? thin? muscular? flabby?

POSTERIOR THORAX: tenderness? masses? *Respiratory excursion:* symmetrical? asymmetrical? no respiratory movements on right/left? subcutaneous emphysema? crepitus? fremitus? estimation of level of diaphragm? spine alignment? tenderness? CVA tenderness? resonance? dull? hyperresonance? diaphragmatic excursion 3–5 cm? comparison of one side to the other? suprasternal notch located? costochondral junctions tender? chest wall stable? vocal fremitus?

LUNG AUSCULTATION: vescular? bronchovesicular? bronchial? whispered pectroliloquy? adventitious sounds? rales? rhonchi? wheezes? crackles? rub? bronchophony? egophony?

BREASTS AND AXILLAE INSPECTION AND PALPATION

BREASTS: male? female? present/absent? color? large? small? well developed? firm? pendulous? flat? flabby? symmetrical/asymmetrical? dimpling? thickening? smooth? retraction? peau d'orange? venous pattern? tenderness? masses? (describe) gynecomastia?

NIPPLES: present/absent? circular? symmetrical/asymmetrical? inverted? everted? pale? brown? rose? extra nipples? discharge? deviation? supernumerary?

AXILLA: shaved/unshaved? odor? masses or lumps? (describe size and shape)

LYMPH NODES: (lateral, central, subscapular, pectoral, epitrochlear) palpable? tender? shotty?

HEART AND PERIPHERAL VASCULAR INSPECTION, PERCUSION, AUSCULTATION, AND PALPATION

HEART: precordial bulge? abnormal palpations? PMI? thrills? heave or lift with pulsation? S_1 loudest at apex? S_2 loudest at base? S_3? S_4? splits? clicks? snap? rub? gallop? *Murmurs:* systolic? diastolic? holosystolic? harsh? soft? blowing? rumbling? grading 1 through 6? high pitch? medium pitch? low pitch? radiating?

CAROTID PULSE: *Note: do not check both right and left carotid pulses simultaneously. Volume:* bounding? forceful? strong? full? weak? feeble? thready? symmetrical? right less than left? left less than right? *Rhythm:* regular? irregular? symmetrical? asymmetrical? bruits present? absent?

APICAL PULSE: record rate; tachycardia? bradycardia? pounding? forceful? weak? moderate? regular/irregular?

PERIPHERAL PULSES: (do not count rate of these pulses except radial) record character, volume, rhythm, and symmetry of brachial, radial, femoral, popliteal, dorsalis pedis, and posterior tibial pulses. *Volume:* full? strong? forceful? bounding? perceptible? imperceptible? weak? thready? symmetrical/asymmetrical? right greater than left? left greater than right? *Rhythm:* regular? irregular? symmetrical? asymmetrical? *Symmetry:* record as symmetrical, right greater than left or left greater than right? Pulse deficit, pulse pressure, BP in both arms, BP lying, sitting and standing if applicable. Jugular venous distention? [record cm above level of sternal angle]

ABDOMEN INSPECTION, AUSCULTATION, PERCUSSION, PALPATION

CONTOUR: irregular? protruding? enlarged? distended? scaphoid? concave? sunken? flabby? firm? flat? flaccid?

SKIN: color; intact? not intact? shiny? smooth? scars? lesions? (describe size, shape, and type of lesion) striae? umbilicus?

BOWEL SOUNDS: present? absent? hyperactive? high-pitched tinkling? gurgles? borborygmus?

PERCUSSION: tympanic? dull? flat? (describe where) liver size 6–12 cm? splenic dullness 6–10th rib? ascites?

PALPATION: splenomegaly? hepatomegaly? organomegaly? masses? aortic pulse? diastasis recti? tenderness? bulges? lower pole of kidneys palpable? inguinal or femoral hernia? inguinal nodes? (describe)

MUSCULOSKELETAL INSPECTION AND PALPATION

BACK: shoulders level? right shoulder higher than left? left shoulder higher than right? alignment? lordosis? scoliosis? kyphosis? ankylosis?

VERTEBRAL COLUMN ALIGNMENT: straight? lordosis? scoliosis? kyphosis?

JOINTS: redness? swelling? deformity? (describe) crepitation? size? symmetry? subluxation? separation? bogginess? tenderness? pain? thickening? nodules? fluid? bulging?

RANGE OF MOTION: describe as full, limited or fixed; estimate degree of limitation; assess range of motion of neck, shoulders, elbows wrists, fingers, back, hips, knees, ankles, toes

EXTREMITIES: compare extremities with each other; describe color and symmetry; temperature: hot, warm, cool, cold, moist, clammy, dry; muscle tone descriptors are firm, muscular, flabby, flaccid. atrophy? fasciculation? tremor?

LOWER EXTREMITIES: symmetry? (describe any variations from normal) abrasions? bruises? swollen? edema? rashes/lesions? (describe) prosthesis? varicose veins?

GENITOURINARY AND RECTUM INSPECTION

RECTUM: hemorrhoids? inflammation? lesions? skin tags? fissures? excoriation? swelling? mucosal bulging? retrocele?

FEMALE GENITALIA: pubic hair distribution and color? nits? pediculosis? lesions? nodules? inflammation? swelling? pigmentation? dry? moist? shriveled, atrophy or full labia? discharge? (describe) odor? asymmetry? varicosities? uterine prolapse? smegma? rash?

MALE GENITALIA: pubic hair distribution and color? nits? pediculosis? circumcised? uncircumcised? phimosis? epispadius? hypospadius? smegma? priapism? varicocele? cryptorchism? hydrocele? swelling? redness? chancre? crusting? rash? discharge? (describe) edema? scrotal sack rugated? atrophy?

NEUROLOGIC

Describe tics, twitches, paresthesia, paralysis, coordination

GAIT: balanced? shuffling? unsteady? ataxic? parkinsonian? swaying? scissor? spastic? waddling? staggering? faltering? swaying? slow? difficult? tottering? propulsive?

ACCESSORY—CN XI: shrugs shoulder? symmetry?

REFLEXES: report as present or absent

COORDINATION: report as to test done

CRANIAL NERVES: may be reported here

MENTAL STATUS

LEVEL OF ALERTNESS: alert? stuporous? semicomatose? comatose?

ORIENTATION: oriented to time, place and person? confused? disoriented?

If confused, check orientation as follows:

Time: ask client year, month, day date.

Place: ask client's residence address, where she/he is now.

Person: ask client's name, birthday.

MEMORY: *Recent memory:* give client short series of numbers and ask client to repeat those numbers later. *Long-term:* ask client to recall some event that happened several years ago.

LANGUAGE AND SPEECH: language spoken? *Speech:* slurred? slow? rapid? difficulty forming words? aphasia?

RESPONSIVENESS: responds appropriately to verbal stimuli? responds readily? slow to respond?

Sample Mental Status Flow Sheet

KEY:
√ Intact
L Limited
D Difficult
∅ Absent

Assessment	Daily						OR	Weekly						OR	Monthly			
	2/1/93		2/2/93		2/3/93			2/1/93		2/8/93		2/15/93			2/1/93		2/1/93	
	A.M.	P.M.	A.M.	P.M.	A.M.	P.M.		A.M.	P.M.	A.M.	P.M.	A.M.	P.M.		A.M.	P.M.	A.M.	P.M.
1. Oriented to person																		
a. First name																		
b. Last name																		
2. Oriented to place																		
a. City																		
b. State																		
c. Name of facility																		
d. Address of facility																		
3. Oriented to time																		
a. Year																		
b. Month																		
c. Date of month																		
d. Day of week																		
f. A.M. or P.M.																		

210

4. Memory														
a. Immediate (minutes)														
b. Recent (days)														
c. Remote (years)														
5. Intelligence														
a. Vocabulary														
b. Calculations														
6. Abstract thinking														
a. Proverbs														
b. Analogies														
7. Mental status test score														
a. MSQ														
b. SPMSQ*														
c. Other														

Source: From Hogstel, M. O.: Assessing mental status, *Journal of Gerontological Nursing* 17(5):43, 1991, with permission.
*See Appendix E.

211

Short Portable Mental Status Questionnaire (SPMSQ)

From Pfeiffer, E.: A short portable mental status questionnaire for the assessment of organic brain deficit in elderly patients. *Journal of the American Geriatrics Society* 23(10):433–441, 1975, with permission.

Instructions: Ask questions 1–10 in this list and record all answers. Ask question 4A only if patient does not have a telephone. Record total number of errors based on ten questions.

+	−	
		1. What is the date today? _____
		Month Day Year
		2. What day of the week is it? _____
		3. What is the name of this place? _____
		4. What is your telephone number? _____
		4A. What is your street address? _____
		(Ask only if patient does not have a telephone)
		5. How old are you? _____
		6. When were you born? _____
		7. Who is the president of the U.S. now? __
		8. Who was president just before him? _____
		9. What was your mother's maiden name? __
		10. Subtract 3 from 20 and keep subtracting 3 from each new number, all the way down.

Total Number of Errors

To Be Completed by Interviewer

Patient's name: _____   Date %_____

Sex: 1. Male   Race: 1. White
     2. Female   2. Black
                             3. Other

Years of education: _____
1. Grade school
2. High school
3. Beyond high school

Interviewer's name: _____

Scoring of the Short Portable Mental Status Questionnaire (SPMSQ)

The data suggest that both education and race influence performance on the Mental Status Questionnaire, and they must accordingly be taken into account in evaluating the score attained by an individual.

For scoring purposes, three educational levels have been established: (1) persons who have had only a grade school education; (2) persons who have had any high school education or who have completed high school; (3) persons who have had any education beyond the high school level, including college, graduate school, or business school.

For white subjects with at least some high school education, but not more than high school education, the following criteria have been established:

0–2 errors	Intact intellectual functioning
3–4 errors	Mild intellectual impairment
5–7 errors	Moderate intellectual impairment
8–10 errors	Severe intellectual impairment

Allow one more error if subject has had only a grade school education.

Allow one less error if subject has had education beyond high school.

Allow one more error for black subjects, using identical education criteria.

Instructions for Completion of the Short Portable Mental Status Questionnaire (SPMSQ)

Ask the subject questions 1 through 10 in this list and record all answers. All responses to be scored as correct must be given by subject without reference to calendar, newspaper, birth certificate, or other aid to memory.

Question 1 is to be scored as correct only when the exact month, exact date, and the exact year are given correctly.

Question 2 is self-explanatory.

Question 3 should be scored as correct if any correct description of the location is given. "My home," correct name of the town or city of residence, or the name of hospital or institution if subject is institutionalized are all acceptable.

Question 4 should be scored as correct when the correct telephone number can be verified, or when the subject can repeat the same number at another point in the questioning.

Question 5 is scored correct when stated age corresponds to date of birth.

Question 6 is to be scored as correct only when the month, exact date, and year are all given.

Question 7 requires only the last name of the president.

Question 8 requires only the last name of the previous president.

Question 9 does not need to be verified. It is scored as correct if a female first name plus a last name other than subject's last name is given.

Question 10 requires that the entire series must be performed correctly in order to be scored as correct. Any error in the series or unwillingness to attempt the series is scored as incorrect.

Apgar Scoring System

	0	1	2
Heart rate	None	< 100	> 100
Respiration	None	Slow or irregular	Cries or makes good effort
Muscle tone	Flaccid	Mild flexion of extremities	Active movement
Reflex response (insert catheter in nostril after clearing oropharynx)	No response	Slow movement or grimaces	Cries, coughs, or sneezes
Color	Blue, pale	Extremities blue, body pink	Completely pink

Pediatric Developmental Milestones

Newborn—should fixate with eyes on objects
  Equal movements
  Responds to noises
2 months—should hold head up 45° when prone
  Social smile
  Coos
4 months—lifts head 90° when prone
  Squeals
  Holds head erect when sitting
  Grasps object
  Follows object 180°
6 months—rolls over to stomach and back
  Reaches for object
  Can sit for few seconds without support
9 months—looks for fallen object
  Feeds self a cracker
  Sits alone
  Transfers object
  Stands holding on
10 months—pulls self to standing
  Plays peek-a-boo

  Says one word
12 months—cruises
12–18 months—walks
  Indicates wants without crying
  Drinks from a cup
18–24 months—Walks backwards
  Feeds self with spoon
  Scribbles
24 months—runs
  Climbs steps
  Draws a vertical line
  Solitary play
3 years—knows first name, age
  Uses plurals in speech
  Draws a circle
  Parallel or interactive play
  Dresses with help
4 years—knows last name
  Separates from parents
  Walks downstairs, both feet alternating
  Interactive games
5 years—dresses alone
  Draws a square
  Follows commands
  Recognizes colors

6–8 years—skips or rollerskates
  Prints numbers, letters
  Can tie a bow
  Defines six words
8+ years—school grade is
appropriate for age

Source: Adapted from Nelms, B., and Mullins, R.: *Growth and Development—A Primary Care Approach*. Prentice Hall, Englewood Cliffs, NJ, 1982, pp. 780–781 with permission.

Fahrenheit and Celsius Scales

F	C	F	C	F	C
500°	260°	203°	95°	98°	36.67°
401	205	194	90	97	36.11
392	200	176	80	96	35.56
383	195	167	75	95	35
374	190	140	60	86	30
356	180	122	50	77	25
347	175	113	45	68	20
338	170	110	43.33	50	10
329	165	109	42.78	41	5
320	160	108	42.22	32	0
311	155	107	41.67	23	− 5
302	150	106	41.11	14	−10
284	140	105	40.56	+ 5	−15
275	135	104	40.00	− 4	−20
266	130	103	39.44	−13	−25
248	120	102	38.89	−22	−30
239	115	101	38.33	−40	−40
230	110	100	37.78	−76	−60
212	100	99	37.22		

$$1.0°F = 0.54°C$$
$$1.8°F = 1.0 \ °C$$
$$3.6°F = 2.0 \ °C$$
$$4.5°F = 2.5 \ °C$$
$$5.4°F = 3.0 \ °C$$

Physical Signs of Malnutrition and Deficiency State*

INFANTS AND CHILDREN

Lack of subcutaneous fat
Wrinkling of skin on light stroking
Poor muscle tone
Pallor
Rough skin (toad skin)
Hemorrhage of newborn, vitamin K deficiency
Bad posture
Nasal area is red and greasy
Sores—at angles of mouth, cheilosis
Rapid heartbeat
Red tongue
Square head, wrists enlarged, rib beading
Vincent's angina, thrush
Serious dental abnormalities
Corneal and conjunctival changes

ADOLESCENTS AND ADULTS

Nasolabial sebaceous plugs
Sores at corners of mouth, cheilosis
Vincent's angina
Minimal changes in tongue color or texture
Red swollen lingual papillae
Glossitis
Papillary atrophy of tongue
Stomatitis
Spongy, bleeding gums
Hyperesthesia of skin
Bilateral symmetrical dermatitis
Purpura
Dermatitis: facial butterfly, perineal, scrotal, vulval
Thickening and pigmentation of skin over bony prominences
Nonspecific vaginitis
Follicular hyperkeratosis of extensor surfaces of extremities

Muscle tenderness in extremities
Poor muscle tone
Loss of vibratory sensation
Increase or decrease of tendon reflexes

Rachitic chest deformity
Anemia not responding to iron
Fatigue of visual accommodation
Vascularization of cornea
Conjunctival changes

*Source: Committee on Medical Nutrition, National Research Council.

Comparison of Joint Diseases*

	Rheumatic Fever	Rheumatoid Arthritis	Osteoarthritis	Gout
Age	Children and young adults	25 and over	Middle and old age	Middle and old age
Sex	Either	Chiefly women	Either	Chiefly men
Cause	Unknown. Autoimmune reaction to streptococci	Unknown. Autoimmune (collagen) disease	Trauma, old age, degenerative changes	Uric acid in blood is increased due to disordered purine metabolism
Joints	Usually large joints, subsiding in one and commencing in another	Multiple, including small joints of hands and feet, usually not axial joints	Usually one large joint (hip, knee, shoulder)	Several

Pyrexia	At onset	In acute stages	None	During acute attack
Permanent deformity	None	Spindle-shaped joints; often gross deformity	Often slight; may be bony enlargement	Deformity mainly from chalky deposits
Heart	Often affected	Infrequently affected	Not affected	Often arteriosclerosis
Treatment	Salicylates; rest in bed. Adrenocortical hormones may be required in acute state	Local heat; physiotherapy; gold; nonsteroidal anti-inflammatory agents; phenylbutazone; indomethacin; analgesics	Analgesics, physiotherapy plus orthopedic measures	Colchicine; probenecid; phenylbutazone; allopurinol; diet

Source: Adapted from Sears, W. G., and Winwood, R. S.: *Medicine for Nurses*, ed. 11. Edward Arnold Publishers Ltd., London, 1970.

227

Dermatomes

DERMATOME

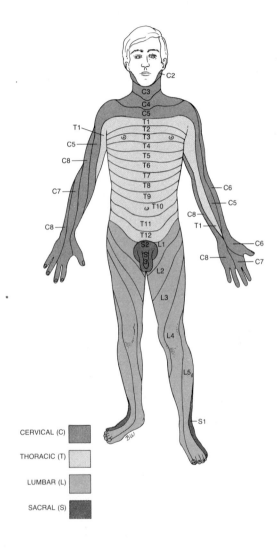

CERVICAL (C)

THORACIC (T)

LUMBAR (L)

SACRAL (S)

Glasgow Coma Scale

Eye Opening	Points	Best Verbal Response	Points	Best Motor Response	Points
Spontaneous Indicates arousal mechanisms in brainstem are active	4	*Oriented* Patient knows who and where he is, and the year, season, and month.	5	*Obey Commands* Do not class a grasp reflex or change in posture as a response.	6
To Sound Eyes open to any sound stimulus	3	*Confused* Responses to questions indicate varying degrees of confusion and disorientation.	4	*Localized* Moves a limb to attempt to remove stimulus	5
To Pain Apply stimulus to limbs, not to face.	2	*Inappropriate* Speech is intelligible, but sustained conversation is not possible.	3	*Flexor: Normal* Entire shoulder or arm is flexed in response to painful stimuli.	4

Never   1

Incomprehensible   2
Unintelligible sounds
such as moans and
groans are made.

None   1

Flexion: Abnormal   3
Slow stereotyped
assumption of decorticate
rigidity posture in
response to painful stimuli

Extension   2
Abnormal with adduction
and internal rotations of
the shoulder and pronation
of the forearm

None   1
Be certain that a lack of
response is not due to a
spinal cord injury.

Source: Adapted from Teasdale, G., and Jennett, B., *Lancet* II, 1974, p. 81; and Teasdale, G., et al. *Acta Neurochirurgica* Suppl. 28, 1979, pp. 13–16.

This scale, originally described in 1974 and further discussed in 1979 by Teasdale and his associates, is widely used in assessing head injury patients, both at the time of the injury and as the patient is observed. The score is recorded every 2 to 3 days.

Height and Weight Tables

1983 METROPOLITAN HEIGHT AND WEIGHT TABLES FOR MEN AND WOMEN ACCORDING TO FRAME, AGES 25–59

Men

Height (In Shoes)*		Weight in Pounds (In Indoor Clothing)†		
Ft.	In.	Small Frame	Medium Frame	Large Frame
5	2	128–134	131–141	138–150
5	3	130–136	133–143	140–153
5	4	132–138	135–145	142–156
5	5	134–140	137–148	144–160
5	6	136–142	139–151	146–164

Women

Height (In Shoes)*		Weight in Pounds (In Indoor Clothing)†		
Ft.	In.	Small Frame	Medium Frame	Large Frame
4	10	102–111	109–121	118–131
4	11	103–113	111–123	120–134
5	0	104–115	113–126	122–137
5	1	106–118	115–129	125–140
5	2	108–121	118–132	128–143

Men		Small frame	Medium frame	Large frame	Women		Small frame	Medium frame	Large frame
5	7	138–145	142–154	149–168	5	3	111–124	121–135	131–147
5	8	140–148	145–157	152–172	5	4	114–127	124–138	134–151
5	9	142–151	148–160	155–176	5	5	117–130	127–141	137–155
5	10	144–154	151–163	158–180	5	6	120–133	130–144	140–159
5	11	146–157	154–166	161–184	5	7	123–136	133–147	143–163
6	0	149–160	157–170	164–188	5	8	126–139	136–150	146–167
6	1	152–164	160–174	168–192	5	9	129–142	139–153	149–170
6	2	155–168	164–178	172–197	5	10	132–145	142–156	152–173
6	3	158–172	167–182	176–202	5	11	135–148	145–159	155–176
6	4	162–176	171–187	181–207	6	0	138–151	148–162	158–179

*Shoes with 1-inch heels.

†Indoor clothing weighing 5 pounds for men and 3 pounds for women.

Source of basic data: *Build Study, 1979*, Society of Actuaries and Association of Life Insurance Medical Directors of America, 1980.

Copyright 1983 Metropolitan Life Insurance Company.

Conversion Rules

To convert units of one system into the other multiply the number of units in column I by the equivalent factor opposite that unit in column II.

	WEIGHT	
I		**II**
1 milligram	—	0.015432 grain
1 gram	—	15.432 grains
1 gram	—	0.25720 apothecaries' dram
1 gram	—	0.03527 avoirdupois ounce
1 gram	—	0.03215 apothecaries' or troy ounce
1 kilogram	—	35.274 avoirdupois ounces
1 kilogram	—	32.151 apothecaries' or troy ounces
1 kilogram	—	2.2046 avoirdupois pounds
1 grain	—	64.7989 milligrams
1 grain	—	0.0648 gram
1 apothecaries' dram	—	3.8879 gram
1 avoirdupois ounce	—	28.3495 grams
1 apothecaries' or troy ounce	—	31.1035 grams
1 avoidupois pound	—	453.5924 grams

VOLUME (AIR OR GAS)

I		II
1 cubic centimeter	—	0.06102 cubic inch
1 cubic meter	—	35.314 cubic feet
1 cubic meter	—	1.3079 cubic yard
1 cubic inch	—	16.3872 cubic centimeters
1 cubic foot	—	0.02832 cubic meter

CAPACITY (FLUID OR LIQUID)

I		II
1 millileter	—	16.23 minima
1 milliliter	—	0.2705 fluidram
1 milliliter	—	0.0338 fluidounce
1 liter	—	33.8148 fluidounces
1 liter	—	2.1134 pints
1 liter	—	1.0567 quart
1 liter	—	0.2642 gallon
1 fluidram	—	3.697 milliliters
1 fluidounce	—	29.573 milliliters
1 pint	—	473.1765 milliliters
1 quart	—	946.353 milliliters
1 gallon	—	3.785 liters

To Convert Celsius or Centigrade Degrees to Fahrenheit Degrees*

Multiply the number of Celsius degrees by $\frac{9}{5}$ and add 32 to the result.

Example: $55°C \times \frac{9}{5} = 99 + 32 = 131°F$

To convert Fahrenheit degrees to Celsius degrees: Subtract 32 from the number of Fahrenheit degrees and multiply the difference by $\frac{5}{9}$.

Example: $243°F - 32 = 211 \times \frac{5}{9} = 117.2°C$

---

*See: *thermometer* for table.

Weights and Measures

APOTHECARIES' WEIGHT

20 grains = 1 scruple   3 scruples = 1 dram
8 drams = 1 ounce   12 ounces = 1 pound

AVOIRDUPOIS WEIGHT

27.343 grains = 1 dram   16 drams = 1 ounce
16 ounces = 1 pound   100 pounds = 1 hundredweight
2000 pounds = 1 short ton   2240 pounds = 1 long ton
1 oz troy = 480 grains   1 oz avoirdupois = 437.5 grains
1 lb troy = 5760 grains   1 lb avoirdupois = 7000 grains

CIRCULAR MEASURE

60 seconds = 1 minute   60 minutes = 1 degree
90 degrees = 1 quadrant   4 quadrants = 360 degrees = circle

CUBIC MEASURE

1728 cubic inches = 1 cubic foot   27 cubic feet = 1 cubic yard
2150.42 cubic inches = 1 standard bushel   268.8 cubic inches = 1 dry (U.S.) gallon
1 cubic foot = about four-fifths of a bushel   128 cubic feet = 1 cord (wood)

DRY MEASURE

2 pints = 1 quart

8 quarts = 1 peck

4 pecks = 1 bushel

LIQUID MEASURE

16 ounces = 1 pint
1000 milliliters = 1 liter
4 gills = 1 pint

4 quarts = 1 gallon
31.5 gallons = 1 barrel (U.S.)
2 pints = 1 quart

2 barrels = 1 hogshead (U.S.)
1 quart = 946.35 milliliters
1 liter = 1.0666 quart

Barrels and hogsheads vary in size. A U.S. gallon is equal to 0.8327 British gallon; therefore, a British gallon is equal to 1.201 U.S. gallons.
1 liter is equal to 1.0567 quarts.

LINEAR MEASURE

1 inch = 2.54 centimeters
12 inches = 1 foot
1 statute mile = 5280 feet

40 rods = 1 furlong
3 feet = 1 yard
3 statute miles = 1 statute league

8 furlongs = 1 statute mile
5.5 yards = 1 rod
1 nautical mile = 6076.042 feet

TROY WEIGHT

24 grains = 1 pennyweight

20 pennyweights = 1 ounce
Used for weighing gold, silver, and jewels.

12 ounces = 1 pound

HOUSEHOLD MEASURES* AND WEIGHTS

Approximate Equivalents: 60 gtt. = 1 teaspoonful = 5 ml
= 60 minims = 60 grains = 1 dram = ⅛ ounce

1 teaspoon = ⅛ fl. oz; 1 dram

3 teaspoons = 1 tablespoon

1 tablespoon = ½ fl. oz; 4 drams

1 tumbler or glass = 8 fl. oz; ½ pint

16 tablespoons (liquid) = 1 cup

12 tablespoons (dry) = 1 cup

1 cup = 8 fl. oz

*Household measures are not precise. For instance, household tsp will hold from 3 to 5 ml of liquid substances. Therefore, do not substitute household equivalents for medication prescribed by the physician.

Patient Positions

POSITIONS

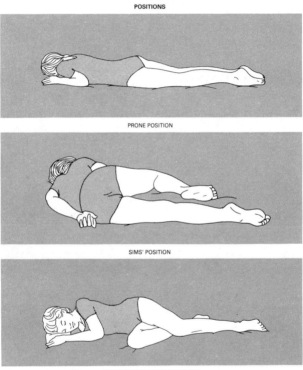

PRONE POSITION

SIMS' POSITION

RIGHT LATERAL RECUMBENT POSITION

POSITIONS

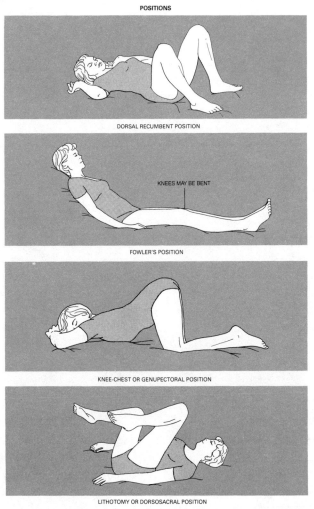

DORSAL RECUMBENT POSITION

KNEES MAY BE BENT

FOWLER'S POSITION

KNEE-CHEST OR GENUPECTORAL POSITION

LITHOTOMY OR DORSOSACRAL POSITION

Glossary

A [P] following a term or an abbreviation signifies that it is particularly pertinent in pediatric assessment. A [G] following a term or an abbreviation means that it is particularly pertinent in geriatric assessment.

accommodation: the ability of the eyes to adapt to viewing objects at various distances

acrochordons [G]: skin tags

acrocyanosis [P]: blueness (cyanosis) of the hands and feet due to slow peripheral perfusion

AC: air conduction

ADL: activities of daily living

adventitious: abnormal breath sounds

AK: above the knee

alopecia: loss of hair of head

A/P: anterior/posterior

arcus senilis [G]: an opaque white ring around the periphery of the cornea (not pathologic)

ascites: serous fluid in abdominal cavity

AV: arteriovenous

B/A: bone/air in Rinne hearing test

BC: bone conduction

BP: blood pressure

borborygmus: gurgling, splashing sound over large intestines

BSE: breast self-examination

bruits: vascular sounds similar to heart murmurs that may be auscultated in areas such as the carotid artery, temple, and epigastrium

capillary hemangioma [P]: a congenital lesion consisting of numerous closely packed capillaries separated by a network of cells

caput succedaneum [P]: an edematous swelling of the scalp caused by pressure

CC: chief complaint, reason client is presenting for care/exam

cephalohematoma [P]: a subperiosteal hemorrhage caused by birth trauma; does not cross suture lines

cerumen: earwax

chloasma: hyperpigmentation, especially of face, commonly associated with pregnancy

clubbing: abnormal enlargement of the distal ends of the fingers and toes, together with curvature of the nails

CN: cranial nerve

CN I: olfactory nerve

CN II: optic nerve

CN III: oculomotor nerve

CN V: trigeminal nerve

CN VI: abducens nerve

CN VII: facial nerve

CN VIII: acoustic nerve

CN IX: glossopharyngeal nerve

CN X: vagus nerve

CN XI: spiral accessory nerve

CN XII: hypoglossal nerve

coloboma: a defect of the pupil of the eye (keyhole pupil)

comedones [P]: blackheads

consanguinity: related by blood

consensual constriction: a reflex action whereby a light beam directed into one eye causes not only the pupil of that eye but also that of the other eye to constrict

crepitus: crackling noise similar to rubbing hair between fingers

CT scan: computed tomography scan.

CVA: cerebrovascular accident; stroke.

C-V: cardiovascular

Cx: cervix

cyanosis: blue-gray color of skin

DES: diethylstilbestrol

diastasis recti: lateral separation of the two halves of the musculus rectum dominis

DOB: date of birth

DIR: deep tendon reflex

Dx: diagnosis

dyspnea: difficulty breathing

dysuria: difficult painful urination

ECG: electrocardiogram

ectropion: eversion of the edge of an eyelid

EDC: expected date of confinement

edema: swelling

encopresis: involuntary discharge of watery feces associated with constipation and fecal retention

ENT: ear, nose, and throat

entropion: inversion of the edge of an eyelid

enuresis: involuntary discharge of urine

EOM: extraocular movement

epistaxis: nosebleed

Epstein's pearls: white-yellow accumulation of epithelial cells on hard palate of newborn

erythema: diffused redness of skin

erythema toxicum neonatorum [P]: a common rash in newborns, characterized by papules or pustules on an erythematous base

excursion (respiratory): of the diaphragm

exophthalmos: abnormal protrusion of eyeball

exudate: accumulation of fluid, pus, or serum or matter that penetrates through vessel wall

FHT: fetal heart tone

fremitus: a vibration palpated or auscultated through the chest wall

G (for gravid): pregnant

genu valgum: knock-knee

genu varum: bowleg

gravity: the number of pregnancies

harlequin sign [P]: a transient redness on one side of the body and paleness on the other; cause unknown

HIV: human immunodeficiency virus

hirsutism: excessive growth of hair in unusual places

hordeolum: inflammation of a sebaceous gland of the eyelid

Hx: history

hypertelorism: abnormal width between two organs, e.g., eyes

hypertropia: abnormal turning of eyes upward

hypotropia: abnormal turning of eyes downward

ICS: intercostal space

jaundice [P]: yellowing of the skin; physiologic jaundice, mild jaundice of the newborn due to functional immaturity of the liver, results in yellowing after the first 24 hours

JVP: jugular venous pressure

keloid: abnormal scar formation

Koplik's spots: small red spots on oral mucosa (sign of measles)

lanugo [P]: fine downy hair on the body of infants, especially premature infants

L & W: living and well

LCM: left costal margin

leukoplakia: formation of white spots or patches on the mucous membrane of the tongue or cheek

leukorrhea: white or yellow discharge from cervical canal or vagina

LICS: left intercostal space

LLQ: left lower quadrant

LMP: last menstrual period

lordosis, kyphosis, scoliosis: swayback, hunchback, lateral curvature of spine

LSB: left sternal border

LUL: left upper lobe

LUQ: left upper quadrant

macule: see lesion list

MCL: midclavicular line

menarche: the onset of menses

metatarsus adductus: adduction of the forefoot distal to the metatarsal-tarsal line

milia [P]: obstructed sebaceous glands, frequently found on the nose and cheeks

mongolian spot [P]: a bluish-black area over the sacral areas of dark-skinned infants

Montgomery's tubercles: lubricating glands on nipples

morphology: structure and form

MRI: magnetic resonance imaging

MSL: midsternal line

nevus flammeus [P]: a circumscribed red, flat lesion found on the face, eyelids, and neck of infants

NG: nasogastric

nuchal: of the neck

nulliparous: without births or pregnancies beyond 20 weeks' gestation (P$\bar{0}$)

nystagmus: constant involuntary movement of eyeball

onychomycosis [G]: a fungus infection of the nails, causing thickening, roughness, and splitting

OD: right eye (L. oculo dextro)

orthopnea: breathing easier in erect position

Ortolani test: test for a congenitally dislocated hip in an infant

OS: left eye (L. oculo sinistro)

OTC: over the counter (i.e., nonprescription)

OU: both eyes (L. oculi unitas)

Pap: Papanicolaou smear

paresthesia: numbness, prickling, tingling

parity: the state of having borne an infant or infants

peau d'orange: dimpled skin condition that resembles the skin of an orange

pectus carinatum: abnormal prominence of the sternum

pectus excavatum: abnormal depression of the sternum

peristalsis: wavelike movements of the alimentary canal

PERRLA: pupils equal, round, reactive to light and accommodation

PI: present illness

pinna: auricle or exterior ear

PMI: point of maximum intensity

polydactyly: abnormal number of fingers and toes

presbycusis [G]: decreased hearing associated with old age

ptosis: dropping of body part (e.g., eyelid)

PVC: preventricular contraction

rales: crackles; added noncontinuous crackling sounds heard on auscultation of the chest; an adventitious sound

RCM: right costal margin

rhonchi: gurgles; added continuous, sonorous, low-pitched sounds heard on auscultation of the chest

Rinne test: a test in which a vibrating tuning fork is used to determine whether a person has normal hearing by comparing the sound perception by tone conduction and by air conduction

RLQ: right lower quadrant

RRR: regular rate and rhythm

RUQ: right upper quadrant

S_1, S_2, S_3, S_4: heart sounds

scaphoid: boat shaped, sunken

Snellen E chart: a wall eye chart

SPF: skin protection factor for sun screens/blocks

STD: sexually transmitted disease

striae: stretch marks, or scarlike breaks in the skin, usually due to stretching of the skin from weight gain

strabismus: a condition in which the optic axes of eyes cannot be directed to same object

syndactyly [P]: fusion of the toes or fingers

thelarche [P]: beginning of breast development at puberty

thrills: palpable heart murmur or rub

tophi: mineral deposits; tartar

TORCH: toxoplasmosis, other (viruses), rubella, cytomegalovirus, herpes (simplex viruses)

TSE: testicular self-examination

turgor: elasticity of skin

UTI: urinary tract infection

vernix caseosa [P]: a white cheeselike substance found in the skin folds of newborns

vertigo: dizziness or lightheadedness

vesicular: pertaining to the alveoli of the lungs

vitiligo: patches of depigmented skin; piebald skin

Weber test for hearing: a test in which a vibrating tuning fork is used to determine which ear is affected by hearing loss

Bibliography

Barry, PD: Psychosocial Nursing Assessment and Intervention. JB Lippincott, Philadelphia, 1984.

Bates, B: A Guide to Physical Examination and History Taking, ed. 5. JB Lippincott, Philadelphia, 1991.

Bowers, AC and Thompson, JM: Clinical Manual of Health Assessment, ed. 2. CV Mosby, St Louis, 1984.

Cella, JH and Watson, J: Nurses' Manual of Laboratory Tests. FA Davis. Philadelphia, 1989.

Eliopoulos, C (ed): Health Assessment of the Older Adult. Addison-Wesley, Menlo Park, CA, 1984.

Kane, RA and Kane, RL: Assessing the Elderly. DC Health Co, Lexington, MA, 1981.

Kempe, C, Silver, H, and Bruyn, H: Handbook of Pediatrics, ed 13. Lange, Los Altos, CA, 1980.

Kozier, B, Erb, G, and Olivieri, R: Fundamentals of Nursing. Addison-Wesley, Menlo Park, CA, 1991.

Malasanos, L, Barkauskas, V, and Stoltenberg-Allen, K: Health Assessment, ed 4. CV Mosby, St Louis, 1990.

Mayfield, PM, Bond, ML, Browning, MA, et al: Health Assessment: A Modular Approach. McGraw-Hill, New York, 1980.

Nelms, B and Mullins, R: Growth and Development: A Primary Health Care Approach. Prentice Hall, Englewood Cliffs, NJ, 1982.

Nelson, M and Mayfield, P: Health assessment. In Hogstel, M: Nursing Care of the Older Adult, ed 2. John Wiley & Sons, New York, 1988, pp. 130–142.

Seidel, H, Ball, J, Dains, J, and Benedict, GW: Mosby's Guide to Physical Examination, ed 2. CV Mosby, St Louis, 1991.

Tanner, JM: Growth at Adolescence, ed 2. Blackwell, Oxford, England, 1962, pp 28–39.

Thomas, C (ed): Taber's Cyclopedic Medical Dictionary, ed 16. FA Davis, Philadelphia, 1989.

Whaley, L and Wong, D: Nursing Care of Infants and Children, ed 3. CV Mosby, St Louis, 1987.

Index

Numbers followed by an "f" indicate figures; numbers followed by a "t" indicate tabular material.